Ida Laudańska-Krzemińska
Quo Vadis, Medicus? Health Behaviour Among Health Professionals and Students

Ida Laudańska-Krzemińska

Quo Vadis, Medicus?

Health Behaviour Among Health Professionals and Students

Managing Editor: Konstantin Kougioumtzis

Associate Editor: Manolis Adamakis

Language Editor: Deirdre Scully

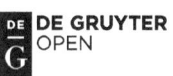
DE GRUYTER
OPEN

Published by De Gruyter Open Ltd, Warsaw/Berlin
Part of Walter de Gruyter GmbH, Berlin/Boston
The book is published with open access at www.degruyter.com.

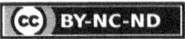
ISBN: 978-3-11-047216-5
e-ISBN: 978-3-11-047217-2

Bibliographic information published by the Deutsche Nationalbibliothek
The Deutsche Nationalbibliothek lists this publication in the Deutsche Nationalbibliografie; detailed
bibliographic data are available in the Internet at http://dnb.dnb.de.

Managing Editor: Konstantin Kougioumtzis
Associate Editor: Manolis Adamakis
Language Editor: Deirdre Scully

www.degruyteropen.com

Cover illustration: © HASLOO

Contents

Introduction

People have always been interested in health and its determinants. For many decades, the number of scientific publications on the determinants of health and disease has increased significantly. Since the early 1970s we have known that our lifestyle largely determines the length and quality of our lives, which has led to an observable increase of interest in health behaviours. The issue is so socially important that it has become one of the most significant topics appearing in the media and popular publications. The average person wants to know more about health, has plenty of opportunities to seek such knowledge (from the internet to the family doctor) and increasingly wants to be sure that this knowledge is evidence-based.

Health professionals are perceived in society as a very important and reliable source of information on health and disease issues. On the other hand, medical treatment often dominates and obscures the role of preventive and promotional activities. The overwhelming obstacle to encouraging such actions (aside from insufficient substantive preparation) is the fact that in medical practice in Poland preventive and promotional activities are not paid for or are paid less by the state. Another significant obstacle may be the lack of consistency between recommendations for successful health behaviour promotion and choices made by health professionals. Physicians, nurses or physiotherapists who do not serve as role models for their patients are much less efficient and, as evidence suggests, they are also less likely to take health promotion actions since they themselves are not fully convinced of the efficacy of such advice.

As a social group, health professionals are representatives of so-called professions of public trust, what translates into their high credibility. This applies particularly to physicians, but other positions held in similar regard are those examined in this study: physiotherapists and nurses. The health condition of the respondents, both during their studies and professional work, has been traditionally considered from the perspective of mental overload, job stress and burnout. Health behaviours and determinants among these socio-economic groups are less frequently the subject of comprehensive analysis. Particularly in the USA and Canada, health behaviours of physicians differ significantly from those of average residents of these countries although not so obviously when compared to individuals of high socio-economic status. Irrespectively, it is postulated that more effort should be made to improve the perception of the medical community by patients in terms of serving as an example (Puddester, Flynn, & Cohen, 2009). This report also indicates areas that require special improvement (e.g. proper diet).

In Poland, there are even fewer studies of this type dedicated to the medical community. Considering the process of transformation in Eastern European countries and the accelerated course in democracy and free market we had to take, certain costs (e.g. health costs) of respective socio-professional group could be expected. Health professionals have been given the opportunity to earn more, to work several jobs and many of them have seized it eagerly. At the same time, these professionals are aware of health determinants and have the relevant knowledge in this area, but a question is whether they can incorporate this knowledge into life. The objective of this study was to describe the strengths and weaknesses of the lifestyle of both the current and future medical staff and to identify some of their subjective determinants.

The author hopes that due to this study's opportunity to "take a look in the mirror" that current and future health professionals will be encouraged to stop and reflect on their own lifestyle and consider the phrase *"Physician Heal Themselves"*. The results of the study may also be considered in the context of preparing health promotion programmes for medical staff.

Furthermore, since most patients believe that "a good doctor is a healthy doctor", the results may also contribute to the formulation of recommendations (already successfully implemented, for example, in the USA and Canada) for the medical community regarding the implementation of a healthy lifestyle, with consideration given to specific challenges faced by health professionals.

1 Health Behaviour and Health Status – What do We Bring to the 3rd Millennium?

Sciences concerned with human health, from medicine to social sciences and the humanities, pay a great deal of attention to human behaviour, treating it as a determinant of health, both in populations and in individuals (Lalonde, 1974; OECD, 2012). At the same time, behaviour is considered to be the most significant factor, which determines health. The intensity of this concern is related to the development of a widely defined concept of health.

To put it simply, the evolution of thought relating to understanding of health has become circular and today we have returned to the roots in a way. In the ancient times body and mind were considered a whole. During illness, natural ways were sought to restore balance between many factors determining health (e.g. Hippocrates' humours) or supernatural powers were invoked (spirits, demons). Similarly, health was treated as a psycho-physical unity (a union of body and mind) in the works of Aristotle and Plato. Often the important role of environmental factors or those related to people's lifestyles was indicated as a condition of good health or recovering health (e.g. Hippocrates emphasised the role of fresh air, exercise, baths, massage and appropriate nutrition). Entirely independent from health concepts of European cultures, around the same time, a naturalist concept of health originated in China. Here too the key to maintain health was the balance between opposite forces determining it, related to human behaviour, emotions and environment. In other words, health was presented as a complex phenomenon, with more or less precisely specified components.

This was followed by a period of dominance of a simple model, reducing health to physiological functions of the body. Its paradigmatic foundation was the Cartesian-Newtonian vision of the world, expressed in duality of soul and matter, body and psyche. This analytical-mechanistic approach introduced many benefits, led to significant progress in medicine and a reduction in numerous health threats (many infectious diseases were contained, death rates in Europe and the United States decreased). This approach had its price, however. Health was perceived from the notion of lack of illness, on which all interest was focused, and basic questions related to causes of illnesses (pathologies, deviations etc.). An illness is mainly limited to its biological dimension and a body is analysed as a machine of its own kind, according to the principles of mechanics. Prevention is addressed mainly to people who are at risk of contracting diseases (e.g. exposed to pathology) and preventative measures concentrate usually on a selected factor. Psychological and social factors are not considered in this approach to health and illness.

Despite everything, changes in the health of populations within developed countries which took place in the last two decades of the 19th century and the first half of the 20th century are called the first health revolution (Healthy People, 1979, p. vii). The main sources of this revolution were: a radical improvement in nutrition, improvement of living conditions, limiting sources of infections by providing clean water and sewage removal, and vaccinations. Evidently this health initiative was effective due to the implementation of widely defined preventative measures, mainly non-medical. People were essentially passive receivers of processes implemented to protect their health.

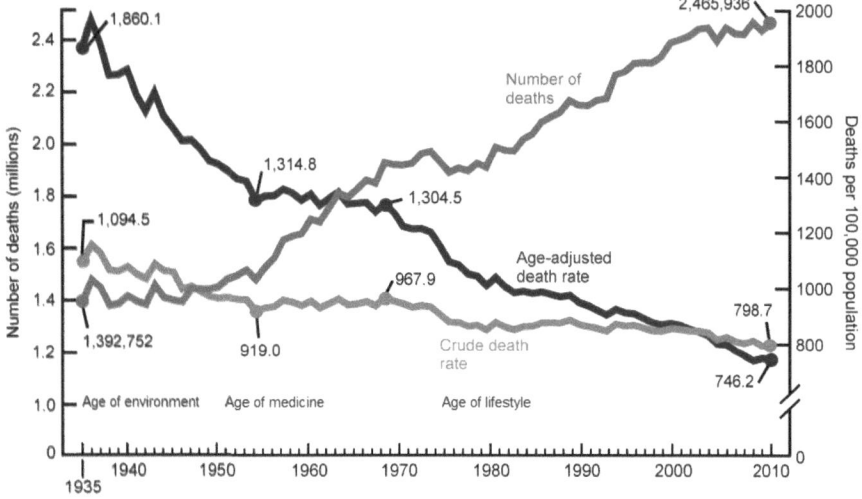

Figure 1.1 Number of deaths, crude and age adjusted rates United States (CDCNCHS, National Vital Statistics Systems, 2010 – modified)

The biomedical model was undoubtedly successful in fighting disease, however its inheritance is organisation of the health care system based on hospitals, clinics and doctors-specialists, with particular emphasis on technological development. As is now evident, the system does not adequately cope with new challenges to public health, including chronic diseases and civilisation-related diseases closely linked to human behaviour and lifestyle. This has been expressed in the US death rate reaching a *plateau*, starting from early 1950s, whereas previously it showed a systematic decrease (see Fig. 1.1).

In the context of the first findings on the impact of behaviour on health, a general hypothesis on behavioural etiology of civilisation-related diseases was formulated and positively verified. According to the Lalonde report, confirmed by subsequent analyses, the most significant factor determining human health is a person's own health-related behaviour, expressed as lifestyle. As a consequence, there is a need for changes in the health care system to deal with this challenge. Medical professionals need new skills to help their patients. This gives rise to a qualitative change in the development of health care, described as the second health revolution (Healthy People, 1979). This marks the beginning of health promotion around the world. Its essence is reflected in a well known slogan *"Your health is in your hands"*, indicating the need for individuals to assume responsibility for their own health. The role of public policy is to create conditions conducive to this. It may be said that we have come a long way from the improvement of hygiene, vaccinations, through fascination with medical technologies, to a return towards people's lifestyle. The age of health promotion is an introduction of various promotional-interventional undertakings in order to strengthen and increase the health potential of the population and a change in social and health policies.

The science and art of health behaviour are eclectic and rapidly evolving; they reflect an amalgamation of approaches, methods, and strategies from social and health sciences, drawing on the theoretical perspectives, research, and practice tools of such diverse disciplines as psychology, sociology, anthropology, communications, nursing, economics, and marketing (Glanz, Rimer, & Viswanath, 2008). In the context of health promotion we will be interested in the social and medical perspectives of human behaviour. Health behaviour, as one of the types of human behaviour, is defined depending on the needs of the science and the paradigmatic orientation of the scientist. The term is used in many sciences (e.g. medical, sociological, psychological sciences) and authors define it or understand it in the way that is most suitable for them.

A particular interest in the studied area concerns the relationships between human behaviour and disease, health and their determinants. Behavioural epidemiology contains two distinguishable concepts which Mason and Powell (1985) clarified. One concept is the epidemiologic relationship between behaviour and disease or health; the other is the epidemiologic study of the behaviour itself and its determinants. For both processes, the means to measure the comparative incidence and prevalence of the behaviour among populations are essential. The first concept is the identification of behaviours that are causally linked to disease and these relationships are complex (Kolbe, 1998). Some behaviours may maintain health, others may threaten it. Some behaviours may have a great influence on the incidence of a given disease whereas others may have a comparatively small influence. Evidence associating some behaviours with certain diseases may be substantial, whereas evidence associating other behaviours with certain diseases may be more tenuous. Some behaviours are more prevalent in a population, others are more rare. Some behaviours must be performed frequently, others need be performed infrequently. Some behaviours have a relatively short incubation period, and thus more immediately may influence prominent health conditions. Other behaviours have a longer incubation period; consequently, the conditions they influence may not have clinical manifestations for 10, 20, or 30 years. Some behaviours may contribute to only one disease, other behaviours may contribute to multiple diseases simultaneously. Some diseases may result from the synergistic effects of multiple behaviours. The results of epidemiologic, biophysical, and clinical research often are combined to test hypotheses about the extent to which various behaviours influence health. The second concept is the application of epidemiologic methods to study the distribution and determinants of behaviours that are causally linked with disease (or health). So this is one step removed from the relationship between behaviour and disease. In terms of smoking, for example, the second component of behavioural epidemiology is the study of who smokes, why they smoke, and, for public health workers, how we can help people to stop smoking or not start.

In the Polish literature one of the first definitions of the studied concept was suggested by Sokołowska (1968), who used a term "medical behaviour" in reference to "behaviour determined by disease or medicine". It was an expression of the contemporary research focus on issues of fighting or overcoming a disease. During the following decade the literature on the subject of understanding health behaviour was extended to include the sphere of health, like in Titkow (1983), *"human actions and activities expressed by means of behavioural variables – related to the sphere of health and disease"*, or in Ostrowska (1980) as, *"a sphere of human actions which refers to health, disease and prevention"*.

Among the definitions of the concept of health behaviour one can indicate those which focus on its behavioural dimension, as in Mackiewicz and Krzyżanowski (1981) who describe it as, *"behaviour considered from the point of view of the significance for health"*, Poździoch (1975): *"any behaviour related to human health"*, or Indulski and Leowski (1971): *"human behaviour such as hygiene habits, following a diet, doing physical exercise in order to strengthen health"*. In Mazurkiewicz (1978) we find a wider perspective relating to cognitive and volitional sphere of human behaviour: *"any behaviour (habits, traditions, attitudes, values recognized by individuals and social groups) in the area of health (...), what a person is like in terms of health is expressed in his or her health behaviour: how they understand health, how they rate it, how they manage it, how they react to other people's health"*. Similarly, Gochman established health behaviour as, *"those personal attributes such as beliefs, expectations, motives, values, perceptions, and other cognitive elements; personality characteristics, including affective and emotional states and traits; and overt behaviour patterns, actions and habits that relate to health maintenance, to health restoration and to health improvement"* (Gochman, 1998, p. 3). On the other hand, Słońska and Misiuna (n.d.) divide the defined actions depending on their perception of the relationships of the undertaken behaviour with health of a person undertaking it. In this way they distinguish health behaviour as, *"any conscious behaviour undertaken by an individual in order to promote, protect and maintain health (irrespective of its consequences)"* and health-related behaviour, which is in their opinion wider and comprises, *"any behaviour (or activity) of an individual which is an element of everyday life and affecting their health"*.

One of the ways of defining health behaviour is by referring it to the objective held by the individual (Korzeniowska, 1997). A classic example of such a systematisation of health behaviour is the proposal suggested by Kasl and Cobb (1966a, b). They distinguished three basic categories of behaviour. *Health behaviour* – denotes those actions undertaken by persons who believe they are well, and who are not experiencing any signs or symptoms of illness, for the purpose of remaining well. This usage confines "health behaviour" to preventive or protecting actions. *Illness behaviour* – comprises those actions undertaken by persons who are uncertain about whether they are well; who are troubled or puzzled by bodily sensations or feelings that they believe may be signs or symptoms of illness; who want to clarify the meaning of these experiences and thus determine whether they are well; and who want to know what to do if they are not. *Sick-role behaviour* – denotes those actions undertaken by persons who have already been designated as being sick, either by others or by themselves. Such behaviours include – but are not limited to – acceptance of a medically prescribed regimen; limitation of activity and of personal, family, and social responsibilities; and actions related to recovery and rehabilitation.

A detailed systematization of health behaviour (by collecting a set of partial definitions) focusing also on the appropriateness of a given behaviour was proposed by Kolbe (1998), who distinguished nine categories (Tab. 1.1). The first six relate to behaviour which affects personal (individual) health of people undertaking it, and the other three relate to behaviour the effects of which affect the health of others.

Table 1.1 A Typology of Health Behaviour (Kolbe, 1998)

Wellness behaviour	any activity undertaken by an individual who believes himself to be healthy for the purpose of attaining an even greater level of health
Preventive health behaviour	any activity undertaken by an individual who believes himself to be healthy, for the purpose of preventing illness or detecting it in an asymptomatic state
At-risk behaviour	any activity undertaken by an individual who believes himself to be healthy but at greater risk than normal of developing a specific health condition, for the purpose of preventing that condition or detecting it in an asymptomatic state
Illness behaviour	any activity undertaken by an individual who perceives himself to be ill, to define the state of his health and to discover a suitable remedy
Self-care behaviour	any activity undertaken by an individual who considers himself to be ill, for the purpose of getting well. It includes minimal reliance on appropriate therapists, involves few dependent behaviours, and leads to little neglect of one's usual duties
Sick-role behaviour	any activity undertaken by an individual who considers himself to be ill, for the purpose of getting well. It includes receiving treatment from appropriate therapists, generally involves a whole range of dependent behaviours, and leads to some degree of neglect of one's usual duties
Reproductive behaviour	any activity undertaken by an individual to influence the occurrence or normal continuation of pregnancy
Parenting health behaviour	any wellness, preventive, at-risk, illness, self-care, or sick-role behaviour performed by an individual for the purposes of ensuring, maintaining, or improving the health of a conceptus or child for whom the individual has responsibility
Health-related social action	any activity undertaken by an individual singularly or in concert with others (i.e., collectively) through organizational, legal, or economic means, to influence the provision of medical services, the effects of the environment, the effects of various products, or the effects of social regulations that influence the health of populations

Another way of defining health behaviour refers to its effects (Korzeniowska, 1997). Health behaviour is considered to be any such behaviour which, in the light of e.g. epidemiological studies, affects the condition of human health (positively or negatively). For example, it includes behaviour which constitutes a risk factor in specific diseases, increasing the risk of developing the disease or death, but also behaviour which strengthens the health potential, is significant for widely defined health, e.g. in accordance with the socioeconomic paradigm. As a result of this approach patterns of behaviour are divided into harmful and beneficial for health. Their examples can be found in the European and national documents outlining the policy and strategy for health: Targets For Health For All, Health 21, Healthy People 2010.

Conceptual, terminological, paradigmatic, methodological diversity related to the use of the concept of "health behaviour" encouraged Puchalski (1989a, 1989b, 1990) to construct a formal diagram to analyse different meanings of the notion. The proposed typology presents three elements, which according to the author are components of each definition of health behaviour: the concept of behaviour (or other related notions, e.g. action, lifestyle), the concept of health (or/and disease, medicine, prevention), the way of linking both concepts. The diversity of adopted meanings of the concept of health behaviour is determined by the third element. Puchalski distinguished two planes describing this relationship: the first one describes the *relationship of behaviour with health* (defined by its direction), the second describes the *area of knowledge* where these relationships are identified.

In the first plane relating to the direction of effect, two basic types of research interest can be distinguished. The effect of *behaviour on health* (behaviour as an independent variable) – this approach is characteristic for medical sciences. Alternatively, we can study the effect of *health on behaviour* (health as an independent variable) – this is the object of interest of social sciences.

In the other plane, relating to identification of behaviour in a specific concept of reality, we can distinguish two areas of research traditionally attributed to two types of science: social and natural. The former area is the sphere of popular awareness; the subject of action decides which behaviour, from his/her point of view, is important for health, the researcher accepts this point of view - this approach is applied mainly in social sciences. The latter area is a reality independent from the popular environment, reflected in scientific concepts and theories. Knowledge is obtained from sources external from the subject of actions - this approach is applied mainly in medical sciences.

By combining the two directions of analysis and individual areas within them we obtain four fields which determine the theoretical perspective or the starting point of theoretical discussion of a scientist (Tab. 1.2). As emphasized by the author of the typology himself, the proposed borders are of conventional and fluid nature and the considered criteria do not exhaust all possibilities in this respect.

Let us try to follow the characteristics of the types of health behaviour definitions distinguished by Puchalski (1989a, 1989b, 1990).

Types I and III include in their scope those forms of activity which a researcher explains while searching for information in popular awareness of a subject (an individual or a group) carrying it out. Group I includes behaviour which a subject describes as determining health, whereas group III includes behaviour which the subject carries out with health in mind (with this intention, for this purpose).

Table 1.2 Typology of health behaviour definitions (Puchalski, 1989a, 1989b, 1990)

	Relationship between behaviour and health	
The area of knowledge:	behaviour and health	health and behaviour
knowledge of the action subject	I	III
knowledge of the action observer	II	IV

Types II and IV include in their scope these forms of activities, a justification for which is searched for by a researcher in the area of codified, objective knowledge e.g. medical, ethical, religious. Group II includes these forms of activities to which science (knowledge the researcher relates to) attributes significant, objective influence on health. Group IV includes behaviour which is the object of interest in various theoretical concepts as an effect of specific health conditions independent of a subject's thinking. Behaviour of this type is often a criterion, an indication for the assessment of health or an element of empirical generalizations describing health-dependent behaviour.

Types of health behaviour distinguished in this way are often not separated and may occur together within specific studies. These distinctions are expressed in systematizations of behaviour made in literature or in ways of defining them. Quite often the discussed concept is defined as any behaviour affecting health, where within its framework behaviour affecting health objectively (the effect of which has been confirmed in scientific studies) and behaviour considered as such in specific social groups are distinguished. In the proposed typology this is behaviour of type I and type II.

Therefore, health behaviour may have both positive and negative impacts on health. It may describe action or refraining from specific actions, it may be carried out consciously or without such an intention, result from beliefs, convictions, family or cultural traditions, popular opinions, specialist academic knowledge, it may be a consequence of availability or popularity of selected actions. In this paper it is assumed, as emphasized by Gochman, that a definition of health behaviour recognizes in addition *"that these personal attributes are influenced by, and otherwise reflect family structure and processes, peer group and social factors, and societal, institutional, and cultural determinants"* (Gochman, 1998, p. 4).

Another issue which is addressed in this paper is health. As we know, the nature of health itself is complex and abstract. A comprehensive definition of health has been adopted by the WHO, however it is not ideal. In health promotion we focus not only on individual heath, but also take a broad look at it. Therefore, health is seen as a resource for everyday life, not an objective of living. Health is a positive concept emphasizing social and personal resources, as well as physical capacities. Therefore, health promotion is not only the responsibility of the health sector, but it goes beyond healthy life-styles to well-being (Ottawa Charter for Health Promotion, 1986). The principles and strategies indicated at global health promotion conferences have evolved. At the 8th Global Conference on Health Promotion in Helsinki they were described as *"Health in All Policies"*, which are constituent parts of countries' contribution to achieving the *United Nations Millennium Development Goals*. They emphasize the responsibility of governments for health and equity, affirm the compelling and urgent need for effective policy coherence for health and well-being and recognize that this will require political will, courage and strategic foresight (The Helsinki Statement on Health in All Policies, 2013).

The belief that health and well-being is a social value, a measure of human development is the basis of the social and health policy of the WHO. The European health policy framework is described in *Health 2020*. In particular, it has to be emphasized that they acknowledge that health challenges are difficult to solve because of their complexity and rapidly changing requirements. The basic strategic objectives are: (1) working to improve health for all and reducing the health divide, (2) improving leadership, and participatory governance for health. In order to achieve the objectives the common policy priorities for health were indicated: (1) investing in health through a life-course approach, empowering people, citizens, consumers, patients to have control over their lives, creating resilient communities; (2) creating healthy, supportive environments for health and well-being; (3) tackling Europe's major health challenges (like non-communicable diseases and communicable diseases); (4) strengthening people-centered health systems, public health capacity and emergency preparedness, surveillance and response (Health 2020). Also the revitalizing role of health staff in this process was indicated. In order to achieve this it is essential to rethink the education of a health professional. This will entail producing a more flexible, multi-skilled workforce to meet the growing challenges in epidemiology, encouraging team based delivery of care, exploring and introducing new forms of service delivery, equipping staff with skills that support patient empowerment, and fostering management and leadership capacities (Health 2020). Inappropriate or problematic health literacy skills of adults in European countries constitute another challenge related to the development of society which has more and more information. It is paradoxical then that patients are faced with challenges related to making healthy lifestyle choices, or choices related to health care, or treatment processes, in which they are by no means prepared or supported. Studies show that weak health literacy competencies are associated with less healthy choices, riskier behaviour, poorer health, less self-management and more hospitalization (Kickbusch, Pelikan, Apfel, & Tsouros, 2013).

2 Psychosocial Determinants of Health Behaviour – Can We Modify the Lifestyle?

We can identify many different determinants of health behaviour and at the same time many different pathways to explore them. Psychologists usually focus on processes within the individual and their research is pursued from the perspective of a cognitive or behavioural theory. Sociologists investigate culture, social structure and relationships within and between societies or social groups. The main interest of medical sciences is human body functions (e.g. physiological processes). Whether engaged in the study of health behaviour at the level of a cell, an individual, or a society, researchers from each field tend to treat their domain as fluid and dynamic. When they do acknowledge the contributions of other domains, they regard these factors as static inputs. As Leventhal, Musumeci and Leventhal (2006) point out, it is possible and necessary to explore the cross-pathway relationships between individual behaviour and social, individual and biological determinants (Fig. 2.1). In this exploration context, collaboration among investigators from different disciplines and integration of different concepts is needed. The outcome would be that we could also get more broadly useful results, especially for health practitioners, lifestyle consultants, health educators, medical specialists or health service managers, social policy.

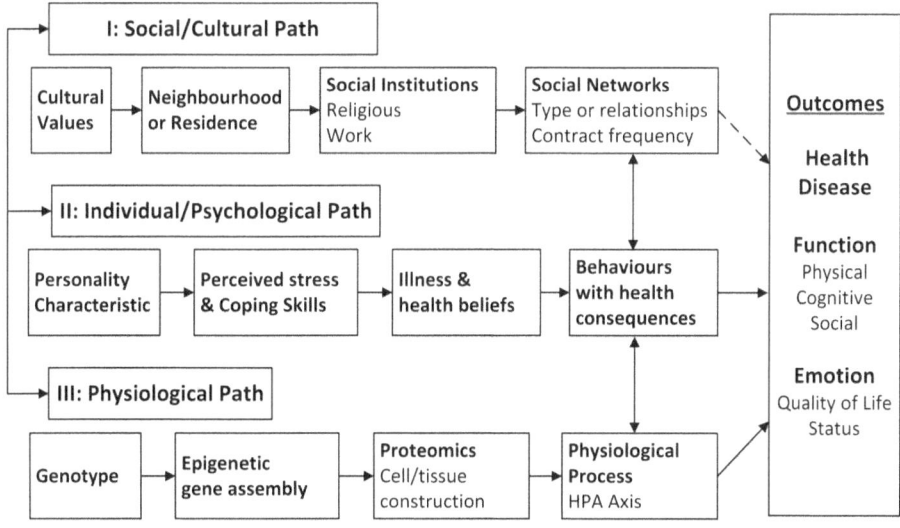

Figure 2.1 Three pathways for the study of health and behaviour (Leventhal et al., 2006)

There are different pathways to study health behaviour and there are also many theories for analysing and predicting health related behaviours. The current study offers a twofold perspective. Firstly, it considers theories as potential ways of explaining health behaviours of current and future medical staff. Secondly, those theories indicate key abilities of health professionals willing to support their patients and clients in changing. We would like to specify the foundations for creating effective intervention programmes, promoting health, in particular in health settings like hospitals, outpatient clinics, medical practices. Psychological theories are probably the most common, these describe the cognitive variables believed to predict behaviour. Cognition is the generic term which refers to organising and evaluating our experiences. Our beliefs, expectations, perceptions, values, motives, and attitudes lead us to interpreting, understanding, filtering and predicting events (Gochman, 1988). There are theories which focus on the individual or intrapersonal level. Three key concepts cut across these theories: (1) behaviour is mediated by cognitions; that is, what people know and think affects how they act; (2) knowledge is necessary for, but not sufficient to produce, most behaviour changes; (3) perceptions, motivations, skills, and the social environment are key influences on behaviour (Theory at a Glance A Guide For Health Promotion Practice, 2005). Common examples of such theories are the Health Belief Model and the Theory of Planned Behaviour (Ajzen, 1991; Becker, 1974; Rosenstock, 1966). These theories are based on the assumption that an individual's activity is the result of evaluating the usefulness of the outcome of the action and probability of achieving it; this will explain whether an individual formulates an intention to change the behaviour. The advantage of those theories consists in their simplicity and precise operationalization (Łuszczyńska & Sutton, 2004). A frequently tested model is the Theory of Planned Behaviour. Ajzen (2002) proposes concrete templates of questions which may be used for various health behaviours, sets of mathematical formulae which enable precise calculation of relations between variables of the model, and thus makes it possible to compare studies. This must have contributed to the popularity of the theory (Łuszczyńska, 2004). At the same time weaknesses of the model relating to the method of its verification are indicated, because in the verifying studies the correlation-regressive pattern prevail (Sutton, 2002) and because during interventions based on this theory, there are rarely manipulated factors building this model (Hardeman, Johnston, Johnston, Bonetti, Wareham, & Kinmonth, 2002).

On the other hand, the essence of the Stages of Change (Transtheoretical) Model (TTM) (Prochasca & DiClemente, 1983, 1992), the Precaution Adoption Process Model (PAPM) (Weinstein, Sandman, & Blalock, 2008) or the Health Action Process Approach (HAPA) (Schwarzer, 2001, 2008) is to explain what causes the behaviour to be initiated and maintained for a long time. They also explain how it can be undertaken to realise the intention of behaviour after a relapse to adverse behaviour and what social and cognitive factors determine maintaining a given behaviour by an individual for a longer time. The first theory, the TTM, assumes a change in behaviour in five stages: precontemplation (the period when an individual has no intention of changing their behaviour), contemplation (an individual considers the pros and cons of undertaking action in the following six months), preparation (an individual makes a decision about intention to act in the following 30 days and prepares to change), action (change in behaviour, undertaking the intended action within less than last six months) and maintenance (stabilization of behaviour and maintaining it for more than six months). Definitions of the stages vary slightly, depending on the behaviour at issue. The model is circular, not linear. Usually, an individual goes through all stages of change in this order, but there is a possibility of relapse to an earlier stage and beginning the process once more or starting the change at any stage. The model has been an object of many studies and has had educational applications, which were particularly readily used in health education for patients/clients who required modification of behaviours such as, smoking, physical activity, or nutrition (Emmons & Marcus, 1994). The advantage of the model is that it presents detailed strategies for individual use (as self-management methods) or for use as part of professional programmes (see Tab. 2.1).

Table 2.1 Educational potential of TTM (Theory at a Glance A Guide For Health Promotion Practice, 2005)

Stage	Definition	Potential Change Strategies
Precontemplation	Has no intention of taking action within the next six months	Increase awareness of need for change; personalize information about risk and benefits
Contemplation	Intends to take action in the next six months	Motivate; encourage making specific plans
Preparation	Intends to take action within the next thirty days and has taken some behavioural steps in this direction	Assist with developing and implementing concrete action plans; help set gradual goals
Action	Has changed behaviour for less than six months	Assist with feedback, problem solving, social support, and reinforcement
Maintenance	Has changed behaviour for more than six months	Assist with coping, reminders, finding alternatives, avoiding slips/relapses (as applicable)

The main objection concerns an artificial division into stages of behaviour and the role ascribed to the two main markers of these stages: expectations of the outcome of action (most important for stage 2) and the sense of one's effectiveness (the role of which increases in subsequent stages) (Łuszczyńska, 2004; Sutton, 2000).

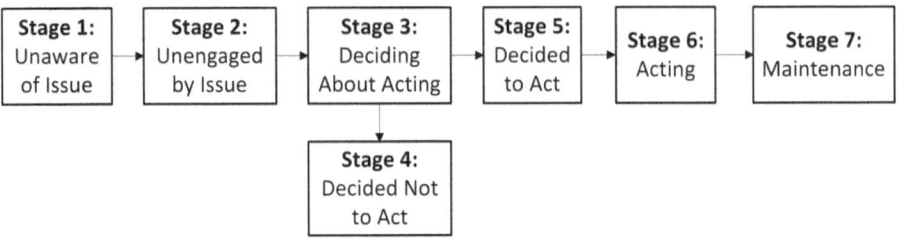

Figure 2.2 PAPM distinct stages (Weinstein et al., 2008)

The PAPM specifies seven distinct stages (see Fig. 2.2), some of which are specific for this model, while others resemble the stages distinguished in the TTM. The author of the model believes that in order to change behaviour effectively an individual must go through all stages of change in the indicated order and that it is not possible to avoid any stage. A relapse to a previous stage is however possible, but once they have completed the first two stages of the model they do not return to them. For example, a person does not move from unawareness to awareness and then back to unawareness (Weinstein & Sandman, 2002). The model appears to be very similar to the TTM, but its particular usefulness in dealing with hazards that have recently been recognized or precaution is emphasized. The PAPM emphasizes the difference between people who are aware of dangers caused by behaviour, but do not undertake it (that is decide not to act) and people who are not aware of specific dangers (in particular new, recently recognized ones). These two groups are faced with different barriers. The PAPM enables health practitioners to develop intervention strategies concentrating on stages preceding making the decision by patients/clients.

The HAPA suggests a distinction between (a) pre-intentional motivation processes that lead to a behavioural intention, and (b) post-intentional volition processes that lead to the actual health behaviour (see Fig. 2.3).

In both stages many social and cognitive variables have been considered, the role of which in the model is varied (discontinuous). The only variable which is significant for both stages is perceived self-efficacy. The authors indicate various possibilities of applying the model in research and interventions pointing out various educational strategies adequate for various stages of change. It is possible to switch from the path-analytic mediator model to a 2-stage model by separating pre-intenders from post-intenders. Moreover, depending on the research question, it is usually a 3-stage model that is chosen (pre-intenders, intenders and actors) which constitutes the best way of reflecting the stage view of the HAPA (Lippke, Ziegelmann, & Schwarzer, 2005).

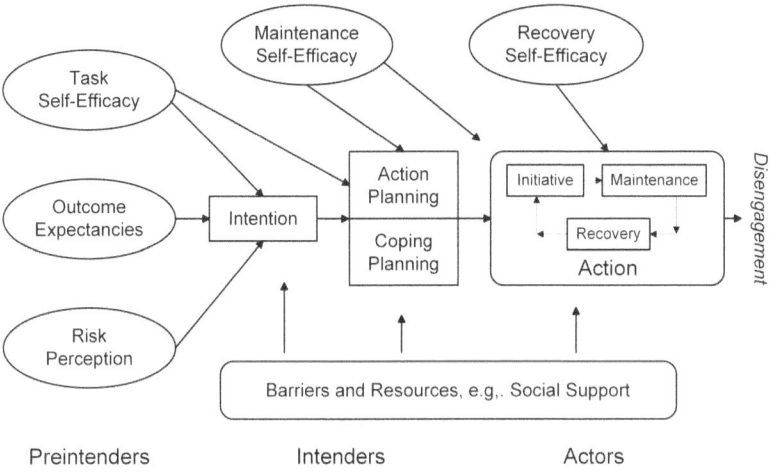

Figure 2.3 HAPA model (Schwarzer, 2008)

The second group of theories include the social context, e.g. Social Cognitive Theory (SCT, Bandura, 1977, 2001). By analyzing behaviour on an interpersonal level we emphasize that individuals are part of and are influenced by social environment. In particular, the emphasis is on the social context of the development of behaviours, related to the influence of people who surround us: family members, teachers, colleagues, health professionals and others through their opinions, advice, support and behaviour. The SCT explains human behaviour as the result of dynamic interaction between personal factors environmental influences and behaviour (Tab. 2.2).

Table 2.2 Educational potential of SCT (Theory at a Glance A Guide For Health Promotion Practice, 2005)

Concept	Definition	Potential Change Strategies
Reciprocal determinism	The dynamic interaction of the person, behaviour, and the environment in which the behaviour is performed	Consider multiple ways to promote behaviour change, including making adjustments to the environment or influencing personal attitudes
Behavioural capability	Knowledge and skill to perform a given behaviour	Promote mastery learning through skills training
Expectations	Anticipated outcomes of a behaviour	Model positive outcomes of healthful behaviour
Self-efficacy	Confidence in one's ability to take action and overcome barriers	Approach behaviour change in small steps to ensure success; be specific about the desired change
Observational learning (modelling)	Behavioural acquisition that occurs by watching the actions and outcomes of others' behaviour	Offer credible role models who perform the targeted behaviour
Reinforcements	Responses to a person's behaviour that increase or decrease the likelihood of reoccurrence	Promote self-initiated rewards and incentives

The main construct explaining the modification of human behaviour proposed by Bandura (1977) is self-efficacy. *"Self-efficacy is the belief in one's capabilities to organize and execute the sources of action required to manage prospective situations"* (Bandura, 1986, p. 391). It is an optimistic belief of an individual in one's capabilities to act according to the chosen objective, irrespective of the obstacles on the way to achieving the objective. Indirectly, self-efficacy affects also the behaviour, influencing the choice of objectives (the stronger the self-efficacy the more ambitious the objectives) and expected gains and losses related to undertaken behaviour (the stronger the self-efficacy, the more gains than losses an individual perceives). In the SCT changeable environmental variables such as barriers and factors facilitating behaviour are also widely considered. The SCT evolved from research on the Social Learning Theory (SLT). The main message of the SLT, so important for health professionals is that people learn not only from their own experience, but also by watching other people's actions and results of these actions. Thus, the educational strategies developed within the SLT and updated in the SCT are so interesting and could be used by health practitioners (see Tab. 2.3). On the other hand, it may be worth considering whether and to what extent health professionals can use modeling in their work and whether their patients would actually benefit.

Table 2.3 Educational potential of SLT (Theory at a Glance A Guide For Health Promotion Practice, 2005)

Concept	Definition	Application
Reciprocal determinism	Behaviour changes result from interaction between person and environment; change is bi-directional	Involve the individual and relevant others; work to change the environment, if warranted
Behavioural capability	Knowledge and skills to influence behaviour	Provide information and training about action
Expectations	Beliefs about likely results of action	Incorporate information about likely results of action in advice
Self-efficacy	Confidence in ability to take action and persist in action	Point out strengths; use persuasion and encouragement; approach behaviour change in small steps
Observational learning	Beliefs based on observing others like self and/or physical results	Point out others' experience, physical visible changes; identify role models to emulate
Reinforcements	Responses to a person's behaviour that increase or decrease the chances of recurrence	Provide incentives, rewards, praise; encourage self-reward; decrease possibility of negative responses that deter positive changes

The third group of theories comprises those focused on ultimate determinants (e.g. macro-system level, sociocultural environment, community level). This group includes Community Organization and Other Participatory Models, which emphasise community-driven approaches to assessing and solving health and social problems. The Diffusion of Innovations Theory (Rogers, 1995) addresses how new ideas, products, and social practices spread within an organization, community or society, or from one society to another. The Communication Theory describes how different types of communication affect health behaviour.

Finally, there are integrative theories that combine all those levels of determinants. Examples of such theories include the Biopsychosocial Model (Irvin & Millstein, 1986; Irwin, Igra, Eyre, & Millstein, 1997), the Bronfenbrenner's Model of Human Development (Bronfenbrenner, 1986) or the Theory of Triadic Influence (TTI) (Faly, Snyder, & Petraitis, 2009). Of all attempts to formulate an integrative theory that predicts health-related behaviours, the TTI appears to be the most comprehensive one (Flay & Petraitis, 1994). The TTI originates from and includes the ideas of Bronfenbrenner and Bandura. The TTI proposes that variables (determinants) can be arranged into three relatively distinct types or "streams of influence": the cultural-environmental stream, the interpersonal social stream and the intra-personal stream (see Fig. 2.4).

Within each stream of influence (personal, social, environmental), two sub-streams are recognized, which can influence behaviour. One is more cognitive/rational in nature, the other is more affective (emotion based). Within each of these streams, three levels of determinants with increasing influence on behaviour are distinguished: ultimate, distal and proximal.

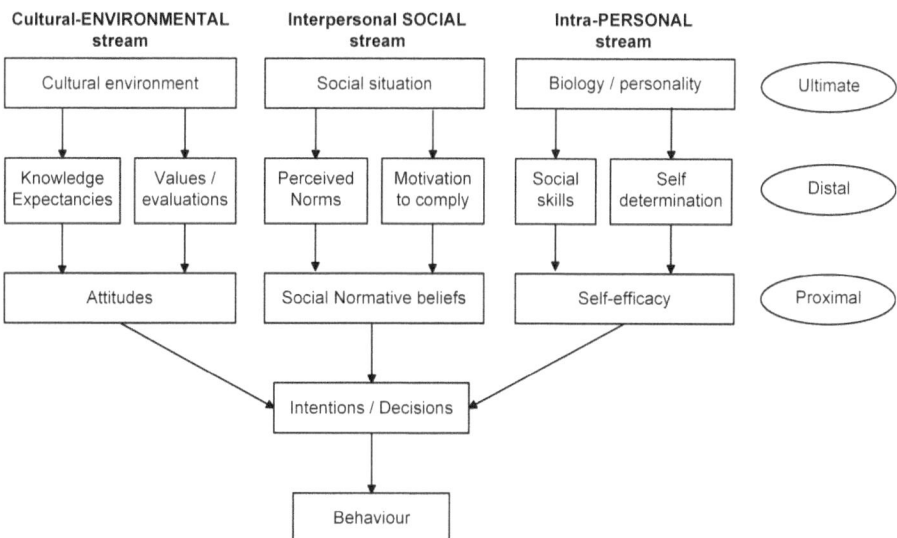

Figure 2.4 Streams of influence in Theory of Triadic Influence (Faly, Snyder, & Petraitis, 2009)

The TTI then proposes that the effects of ultimate and distal causes of behaviour flow predominantly within each stream (personal, social and environmental factors) and act through a small set of proximal predictors of behaviour (e.g. self-efficacy, social normative beliefs, attitudes and intentions), with multiple mediating factors between (Fly, Snyder, & Petraitis, 2009). Proximal causes are usually most influential, in particular in relation to a single specific behaviour (for example, beliefs concerning specific health behaviour, perceived personal health risks, perceived subjective norms of peers or parents, self-efficacy). Distal causes have indirect effects on behaviour. They are related to social relations, knowledge and the system of values, social competence (e.g. internal locus of control, self-esteem, the perceived behaviour of significant others, the parent-child relationship) and have weaker direct effect on single behaviour than proximal determinants, thus their effects on behaviour are mediated by another, more proximal, factor. The ultimate causes are more deeply rooted and less predictive of behaviour than distal and proximal determinants. They are believed to be almost unchangeable (like personality, Social Economic Status, religiousness) (Fly, Snyder, & Petraitis, 2009).

Increasingly often co-occurring health-related behaviour is identified (Allegrante, Peterson, Boutin-Foster, Ogedegbe, & Charlson, 2008; Fine, Philogene, Gramling, Coups, & Sinha, 2004; Pronk, Anderson, Crain, Martinson, O'Connor, Sherwood, & Whitebird, 2004). Hence, factors related to such clusters are sought. The TTI is a model which allows for searching for them. If such factors exist, then there would be support for the development of more integrated approaches to promoting healthier lifestyles. As predicted by Prochaska (2008) *"Multiple Health Behaviour Research represents the future of preventive medicine"* (p. 281).

Using the TTI model Wiefferink, Peters, Hoekstra, Dam, Buijs and Paulussen (2006) identified several protective determinants in adolescents: living with supportive parents, high self-esteem, high perceived personal health risk, perceived healthy behaviour of peers and parents, and perceived acceptability of the healthy behaviour by peers and parents. However, adolescents can be seduced into unhealthy behaviour by the immediate gratification they anticipate. Dusseldorp's and colleagues (2014) findings suggest that addressing self-control and descriptive norms of friends might reduce a broad range of negative behaviours. They also highlight that parental monitoring and descriptive norms of parents may remain important ultimate targets for intervention development, since these provide good opportunities for achieving positive health outcomes sustainable for life. These findings have broadly educational consequences. This identifies the direction in which health educators should look for a more efficient programme design. There are recognized, potentially modifiable distal determinants (as opposed to ultimate determinants like personality), which may become an object of interventions including many various health behaviours (Wiefferink, Peters, Hoekstra, Dam, Buijs, & Paulussen, 2006).

3 Health Behaviour of Health Professionals – What Should it Be Like?

Health behaviours are some of the well-known and well documented factors affecting health. From classic large studies in Framingham in the USA to another study in Alamenda County in California (Housman & Dorman, 2005; Levy & Wang, 2013) such behaviour as physical activity, appropriate nutrition, moderate alcohol drinking and non-smoking were clearly demonstrated as key for the risk of developing circulatory system diseases and better health indicators in general. However, more detailed studies of links between health behaviour and health do not always give unequivocal results. This may result from various relationships between behaviours. Gniazdowski (1990) indicates that developing a condition with a behavioural basis is determined by the number, nature, intensity and interaction of behavioural factors of a person. The interaction of these factors may be additive in nature – which means adding up the influences of individual risk factors of a condition. The probability of developing a condition increases proportionally with the weight of individual risk factors of a given person. Another type of interaction is a synergistic effect, which means additional intensification of the effects of one risk factor by the presence of another (smoking tobacco by people working with asbestos). The opposite effect is also possible when one behaviour neutralizes the negative impact of another behaviour on health (a diet rich in green vegetables decreases a negative effect of smoking on health).

McGinnis and Foege (1993) have identified the non-genetic factors that increased total mortality in the United States and estimated their contributions to the ten leading mortality diagnoses: (1) tobacco use, (2) inadequate or excessive nutrition (dietary habits), (3) inadequate aerobic exercise, (4) excessive alcohol consumption, (5) lack of immunization against microbial agents, (6) exposure to poisons and toxins, (7) firearms, (8) risky sexual behaviours, (9) motor vehicle trauma, (10) use of illicit drugs. The majority of diseases and causes of deaths in developed countries (cancer, heart disease, stroke etc.) are attributed to co-occurring health behaviours such as smoking, alcohol abuse, physical inactivity, poor diet. There is evidence that unhealthy behaviours co-occur and as a result increase the risk of developing the disease. Analysis of data from the 2001 National Health Interview Study indicated that the majority of adults in the United States met criteria for two or more risk behaviours (Fine, Philogene, Gramling, Coups, & Sinha, 2004; Pronk, Anderson, Crain, Martinson, O'Connor, Sherwood, & Whitebird, 2004). The consequences of an increasing number of risk factors identified in patients are of a medical, but also a financial nature (Edington, Yen, & Witting, 1997). Longitudinal data indicate that effectively treating two behaviours reduces medical costs by about $2,000 per year (Edington, 2001). Undertaking actions in the area of multiple risk behaviours offers a chance of potentially greater health benefits, maximizes the use of means and resources related to health promotion, and decreases the costs of health care.

This book analyses these four basic health behaviours which are the main risk factors of lifestyle-related diseases: physical activity, nutrition, alcohol consumption and smoking. They are described below in the context of their relations to health and the resulting recommendations.

3.1 Physical Activity

Physical activity is one of the key components in a healthy way of life. Physical activity, which is defined as, "bodily movement that is produced by the contraction of skeletal muscle and that substantially increases energy expenditure" (US Department of Health and Human Services, 1996, p. 20), or, "any force exerted by skeletal muscles that results in energy expenditure above resting level" (Caspersen, Powell, & Christensen, 1985, p. 127), has been fundamentally restricted through changes to society throughout the 20th century. Physical activity can take many forms and consist of miscellaneous activities, such as occupational, household, transport, and leisure-time activities. Similar to other health behaviours, physical activity is conditioned by socio-demographic factors. The Special Eurobarometer Research (2014) has shown that the number of people (in Europe) who never exercise or engage in sport increased by 3% within the previous five years. A similar increase has been registered in Poland. Approximately 35% of Polish people do not willingly engage in daily physical activities, e.g. bike riding, gardening, dancing etc. which is greater than the EU-average of 30% inactive (Special Eurobarometer Research, 2014). In Europe we can see that the percentage of people not engaging in vigorous physical activities has increased by 4%, to an overall of 54%, within a decade. In Poland the overall percentage is even greater at 59%. The percentage of Europeans not doing moderate physical activity has increased to 44%. Poles seem especially loath to this kind of physical activity with 56% not doing it at all. In Europe we see a beneficial change regarding daily walking. Unfortunately, in comparison to the European norm, Poles appear unfavorable as they are less likely to have walked for ten or more minutes on at least four days (41% Poles compared to 60% percentages for Europe). In Poland we have also the highest proportion of respondents (25%) who not walk for ten minutes or more per day during a week, in comparison to 13% for Europe. Poles' physical activity decreases with age, but increases with better education and better financial self-assessment (Aktywność fizyczna Polaków, 2013). Poles most often do sport for health (70%) and pleasure (61%). There is a connection between the reasons for doing sport and the choice of sport or physical activity. Running, swimming, cycling, aerobics and fitness are chosen by people who prefer to do the sport for health reasons. Exercise at the gym and bodybuilding are also selected for health, but also to enhance body-image. On the other hand, enjoyment is the main reason given for dancing, hiking, playing soccer, doing winter sports and volleyball.

The observed changes in physical activity result especially in deteriorating health indicators. As a basic component of energy expenditure physical activity has a huge impact on the energy balance and body composition. One of the particularly important health results which can be achieved, is the substantial reduction in abdominal subcutaneous and visceral fat (McArdle, Hillman, Beilin, & Watts, 2007). Aerobic exercise, especially, longer and more prolonged is consistent with the increase of high density lipoprotein (HDL) cholesterol (Durstine, Grandjean, Cox, & Thompson, 2002). There is substantial evidence that physical activity is an effective method of enhancing insulin sensitivity and therefore counteracting insulin resistance (Hardman & Stensel, 2003). Physical activity is also well-known as the main, modified risk factor with medical disturbances such as: cardiovascular disease (CVD), coronary heart disease, stroke, type 2 diabetes, osteoporosis, colon and breast cancers, possibly of endometrial and prostate cancers (Buttriss & Hardman, 2005; Department of Health, 2004; Gonçalves, Florêncio, de Atayde Silva, Cobucci, Giraldo, & Cote, 2014; Langsetmo, Hitchcock, Kingwell, Davison, Berger, Forsmo, Zhou, Kreiger, & Prior, 2012; Miles, 2007; Physical Activity Guidelines Advisory Committee, 2008; Schmid & Leitzmann, 2014; Warburton, Charlesworth, Ivey, Nettlefold, & Bredin, 2010; Warburton, Nicol, & Bredin, 2006; WHO, 2010). Physical activity and exercise can decrease the risk of fractures and injurious falls (Pereira, Baptista, & Infante, 2014; Thibaud, Bloch, Tournoux-Facon, Brèque, Rigaud, Dugué, & Kemoun, 2012). Scientific research supports the observation that physical activity has a positive impact on the mental health. The release of endorphins (endogenous opioids) in the brain can lead to mood enhancement (Peluso & Guerra de Andrade, 2005). Motor skills training can also improve the executive functions of cognition (Dishman, Berthoud, Booth, Cotman, Edgerton, Fleshner, & Zigmond, 2006; Chien-Ning, Bih-Shya, Meei-Fang, 2011). Physical activity is linked to a better healthier quality of life, general well-being, as well as self-esteem (Anokye, Trueman, Green, Pavey, & Taylor, 2012; Maher, Doerksen, Elavsky, Hyde, Pincus, Ram, & Conroy, 2013; Sonstroem, 1984). Exercise has been shown to help reduce the risk of depression (Dinas, Koutedakis, & Flouris, 2011). Physical activity has a major health effect worldwide. Generally, regular physical activity increases life expectancy (Lee, Shiroma, Lobelo, Puska, Blair, & Katzmarzyk, 2012; Reimers, Knapp, & Reimers, 2012).

Suggestions regarding physical activity and exercise recommendations are quite varied (Blair, LaMonte, & Nichaman, 2004). The most popular recommendation during the 70s and 80s, provided by the American College of Sports Medicine (ACSM), concentrated on improvement and maintenance of physical fitness. The result was that many people were not able to live up to these recommendations. It was also believed that this inability did not benefit health. From 1990 onwards ACSM noticed the beneficial effects of frequent exercise done for longer duration, but at a lower intensity than earlier prescriptions. This was the beginning of a paradigm that includes activity recommendations for both performance and health-related outcomes (Blair, LaMonte, & Nichaman, 2004). Table 3.1 shows the summary of current suggestions and recommendations from leading health agencies regarding required physical activity.

Table 3.1 Current PA recommendation for adults of American College of Sports Medicine, WHO, CDC

	Frequency	Duration	Intensity	Additional indications
WHO EU region[1]	≥5 wk⁻¹	≥30 min	moderate-intensity aerobic activity	muscular strength training 2-3 days per week · possible accumulation bouts of at least 10 minutes duration
	≥3 wk⁻¹	≥20 min	vigorous-intensity aerobic activity	
	≥5 wk⁻¹	any combination of walking, moderate- or vigorous-intensity activities ≥ 600 METs per week		
WHO global recommendation[2] CDC[4]	≥150 min per week		moderate-intensity	muscle-strengthening activities ≥ 2 days per week · possible accumulation bouts of at least 10 minutes duration
	≥75 min per week		vigorous-intensity aerobic activity	additional health benefits, increase their moderate-intensity aerobic physical activity to 300 min per week, or to 150 min of vigorous-intensity aerobic physical activity per week, or an equivalent combination of moderate- and vigorous-intensity activity
	equivalent combination of moderate- and vigorous-intensity aerobic activity			
ACSM[3]	5 d·wk−1	≥30 min·d⁻¹ total ≥150 min·wk⁻¹	moderate-intensity cardiorespiratory exercise training	2-3 d·wk⁻¹, resistance exercises for each of the major muscle groups, and neuromotor exercise involving balance, agility, and coordination. ≥2 d·wk⁻¹ flexibility exercises for each the major muscle-tendon groups (a total of 60 s per exercise) · possible accumulation bouts of at least 10 minutes duration
	≥3 d·wk⁻¹	≥20 min·d⁻¹ ≥75 min·wk⁻¹	vigorous-intensity cardiorespiratory exercise training	
	combination of moderate- and vigorous-intensity exercise to achieve a total energy expenditure of ≥500-1000 MET·min·wk⁻¹			

[1] - Country profiles on nutrition, physical activity and obesity in the 53 WHO European Region Member States. Methodology and summary, WHO 2013; EU Physical Activity Guidelines Recommended Policy Actions in Support of Health-Enhancing Physical Activity 2008; http://ec.europa.eu/sport/library/policy_documents/eu-physical-activity-guidelines-2008_pl.pdf

[2] - Global recommendations on physical activity for health., WHO 2010.

[3] - Garber et.al.2011; American College of Sports Medicine. ACSM's Guidelines for Exercise Testing and Prescription. 8th ed. Philadelphia (PA): Lippincott Williams & Wilkins; 2010. p. 366.

[4] - http://www.cdc.gov/physicalactivity/everyone/guidelines/adults.html

As can be seen, the recommendations regarding healthy physical activity are similar and can easily be integrated into an adult's work schedule and free time. Such a consensus has been made possible due to equivalent results in regard to the connection between the weekly physical activity and lifestyle diseases. On the other hand, results regarding the amount of dose accumulation are not equivalent, therefore the recommendations are more flexible. At the same time, muscle-strengthening training is listed in every recommendation as a complementary point and not merely a suggestion, the same applies for flexibility exercises. European Union countries, including Poland, are keen to increase the physical activity of inhabitants. Over the past decade an intense monitoring and consistent social policy has been taking place which promotes good practical solutions and encourages member states to incorporate the proposed solutions (Council conclusions on nutrition and physical activity, 2014; Green Paper, 2005; Physical activity and health in Europe, 2006). Health-care professionals are one of the key components of this policy, not only as beneficiaries, but more importantly as executors.

3.2 Nutrition

Nutrition is an important determinant of health. Research studies have revealed that there is an consistent relationship between unhealthy diet and the emergence of a range of chronic non-infectious diseases, including cardiovascular diseases, various cancers, and diabetes mellitus (Brunner, Mosdøl, Witte, Martikainen, Stafford, Shipley, & Marmot, 2008; Heidemann, Schulze, Franco, van Dam, Mantzoros, & Hu, 2008; Isharwal, Misra, Wasir, & Nigam, 2009; Kant, 2004; Nettleton, Polak, Tracy, Burke, & Jacobs, 2009; Panagiotakos, Pitsavos, Chrysohoou, Palliou, Lentzas, Skoumas, & Stefanadis, 2009). In the past decade, the growing interest in nutrition epidemiology has been concentrated on the investigation at the level of foods and dietary patterns and less on investigations at the level of individual nutrients (Hu, 2002; Kant, 2004; Nettleton, Schulze, Jiang, Jenny, Burke, & Jacobs, 2008). Such an approach gives a better picture of the complex impact of the general diet on health than an analysis of a single food item only.

The correlations between the recommended consumption of particular food groups and health conditions are well known. The proper consumption of **vegetables and fruits** is associated with reduced risk for cardiovascular disease (Hooper, 2007), heart disease (He, Nowson, Lucas, & MacGregor, 2007), stroke (Dauchet, 2005), hypertension (Svetkey, Simons-Morton, Vollmer, Appel, Conlin, Ryan, Ard, & Kennedy, 1999), many cancers (World Cancer Research Fund/American Institute for Cancer Research, 2007), vision problems associated with aging (Cho, 2004), possibly diabetes (Montonen, 2005), and weight reduction (National Center for Chronic Disease Prevention and Health Promotion, 2007). Additionally, the consumption of **legumes** decreases total and LDL cholesterol and other risk factors for heart disease

(Bazzano, 2011; Mattei, Hu, & Campos, 2011). Legume fiber was among the fiber types associated with reducing risk for metabolic syndrome (Hosseinpour-Niazi, 2011). Eating legumes or beans especially may reduce the risk for developing certain types of cancers (Amarowicz, 2008; Cade, 2007; Dahm, 2010; Kolonel, 2000; Thompson, 2012; Wang, 2011).

The highest category of **whole grain** intake is associated with a 21% reduction in cardiovascular disease risk, a 26% lower risk of type 2 diabetes and consistently less weight gain. Higher levels of whole-grain intake are associated with lower levels of fasting glucose, total and LDL - cholesterol, systolic and diastolic blood pressure, and weight gain (Ye, Chacko, Chou, Kugizaki, & Liu, 2012). The German Nutrition Society ranked the evidence on whole grains and health and determined that there is convincing evidence that the whole grain consumption reduces total and LDL cholesterol, probable evidence that it reduces the risk to type 2 diabetes, possible evidence that it reduces the risk of obesity in adults, but insufficient evidence that it reduces the risk of metabolic syndrome (Hauner et al., 2012). A regular consumption of three or more food portions per day based on wholegrain cereals decrease the risk of CVD, and the risk of type 2 diabetes by 20-30%. Protection against the risk of colorectal cancer and polyps, other cancers of the digestive tract, cancers related to hormones and pancreatic cancer have been associated with the regular consumption of wholegrain cereals and derived products (Gil, Ortega, & Maldonado, 2011).

Pan, Sun, Bernstein, Schulze, Manson, Willett and Hu (2011) suggest that **red meat** consumption, particularly processed red meat, is associated with an increased risk of type 2 diabetes. They also estimated that substitutions of one serving of nuts, low-fat dairy, and whole grains per day for one serving of red meat per day are associated with a 16–35% lower risk of type 2 diabetes. The findings from a Swedish prospective cohort of men and women indicate that processed meat consumption is positively associated with risk of stroke (Larsson, 2011a, b) and the results from meta-analysis indicate that consumption of fresh red meat and processed red meat as well as total red meat is associated with increased risk of total stroke and is chemic stroke, but not hemorrhagic stroke (Kaluza, Wolk, & Larsson, 2012). The results from the European Prospective Investigation into Cancer and Nutrition support a moderate positive association between processed meat consumption and mortality, in particular due to cardiovascular diseases, but also to cancer (Rohrmann et al., 2013). There is more evidence that high consumption of red meat, particularly processed meat may be a risk factor for coronary heart disease, the metabolic syndrome, some types of cancers, whereas white meat may be associated with reduced risk of chronic liver disease and hepatocellular carcinoma as well as with the decrease of men's death rate (Freedman et al., 2010; Kappeler, Eichholzer, & Rohrmann, 2013; Micha, Wallace, & Mozaffarian, 2010; Sinha, Cross, Graubard, Leitzmann, & Schatzkin, 2009; Smolinska & Paluszkiewicz, 2010). On the one hand **Fish** consumption has the advantages listed below, but on the other hand it also presents risks. Due to increased exposure to toxicants in fish, such as methylmer cury (MeHg) and polychlorinated biphenyls (PCBs), it is recommended to limit fish consumption in risk groups (U.S. Environmental Protection Agency (EPA), 2004). Nevertheless, many organizations of physicians and nutritionists encourage fish consumption for the entire population as a way to increase dietary intake of the n-3 (omega-3) long chain polyunsaturated fatty acids (LCPUFAs) that may prevent cardiovascular disease, risk of fatal ischemic heart disease, risk of stroke and improve neurological development (Breslov, 2006; Kris-Etherton, Harris, & Appel, 2002; Kris-Etherton & Innis, 2007; Larsson & Orsini, 2011; Lee et al., 2009; Mozaffarian, 2011). Fish consumption is also associated with decreased risk of depression for women, but it also moderately protects from cerebrovascular risk (Chowdhury et al., 2012; Smith, Sanderson, McNaughton, Gall, Dwyer, & Venn, 2014). Fish consumption is considered one of the key components of a cardioid-protective diet. Current cardiovascular guidelines for healthy individuals encourage consumption of a variety of fish, preferably oily types, at least twice a week. (Gidding et al., 2009; Graham et al., 2007). However it is necessary to have a reliable, comprehensive information which consider the different aspects of consumer choice regarding fish. Advice regarding this topic should consider the following challenges: toxicological hazards, nutritional benefits, environmental sustainability, economic influences (Oken et al., 2012).

Meeting and exceeding recommendations for consumption of **dairy products** each day leads to better nutrient status, can lead to improved bone health, and is associated with lower blood pressure and a reduced risk of cardiovascular disease and type 2 diabetes (Rice, Quann, & Miller, 2013). The observational evidence does not support the hypothesis that dairy fat or high-fat dairy foods contribute to obesity or cardiometabolic risk, and suggests that dairy or high-fat dairy consumption within typical dietary patterns is inversely associated with obesity risk, cardiovascular disease risk, heart disease, stroke or diabetes (Elwood, Pickering, Givens, & Gallacher, 2010; Fumeron et al., 2011; Kratz, Baars, & Guyenet, 2013; Rice, Quann, & Miller, 2013; Soedamah-Muthu et al., 2011).

In terms of **fat** intake the best health results, which are related to the decrease of coronary heart disease risk; can be given by replacing trans- or saturated fat with poly- and monounsaturated fat (Hu, Stampfer, & Manson, 1997; Willett, 2012). There is also well know protective role for high olive oil consumption on the risk of CVD, stroke and type 2 diabetes (Ruiz-Canela & Martínez-González, 2011; Salas-Salvadó, 2011; Samieri, 2011).

Proper nutrition pyramids are currently the most popular, complementary and socially recognizable summaries in regard to the correct nutrition. The first version of such a pyramid was presented in 1992 by the U.S. Department of Agriculture (USDA) under the title, *The Food Guide Pyramid*; the latest version of nutrition pyramid, dated 2005, is different in both design and recommendations and is known by the name *MyPyramid*. Its recommendations were subsequently transcribed into a form called *MyPlate*. They are based on *Dietary Guidelines for Americans 2010* (USDA, 2010). A proper nutrition pyramid has also been proposed by Walter Willet from the Harvard School of Public Health (U.S.) in 2003, (updated in 2008 to *Healthy Eating Pyramid*). In 2011 they also created the *Healthy Eating Plate* based on the best available scientific evidence of the links between diet and health. The main task of the authors is the correction of previous mistakes – in their opinion – in the USDA food pyramid and plate (Willet & Stampfer, 2006). The Polish Institute of Nutrition and Food located in Warsaw has also developed and is promoting nutritional rules in the form of a pyramid (Principles of Proper Nutrition, 2009). All of these pyramids have in common that physical activity is one of the most important elements of a healthy lifestyle associated with the amount and quality of the consumed food. Diet, which is appropriately balanced through physical activity, can maintain the normal body weight and helps to have the strength and energy for daily challenges. Golden Chart of Property Nutrition is another document which includes guidelines regarding a balanced diet and it belongs to the consensus of Polish organizations dealing with the promotion of healthy lifestyle (Golden Chart of Property Nutrition, 1997). The following diet recommendations are promoted in Polish documents: whole grain cereal products at every meal, as well as vegetables and fruits; and between the meals a minimum of two cups of milk (best light) or yogurt, kefir as well as 1 – 2 slices of cheese, one portion of fish, poultry, peas, beans or meat, one tablespoon of oil or olive oil, and two teaspoons of light margarine (without trans fats), a minimum of one litre mineral water and natural vegetables/fruits juices, minimum three moderate meals per day, but absolutely including breakfast. Salt, sugar, and alcohol should be limited. These recommendations are the development-base for research which examines the dietary patterns of health students and professionals. There are also specially-developed recommendations for medical staff relating to their health and well-being, which emphasise the challenges of physicians' diets at work (Puddester, Flynn, & Cohen, 2009). Some of the most important suggestions include eating breakfast, taking healthy and convenient snacks, planning and prioritizing nutritious breaks, preparing a balanced nutritional intake, analysing and recognising the emotional and physical symptoms indicating that it's time to eat and drink, building a healthy environment for nutritional behaviour at work.

3.3 Smoking

Almost 6 million people die from tobacco use each year, both from direct tobacco use and second-hand smoke. By 2030, this number will increase to 8 million, accounting for 10% of all deaths (Tobacco fact sheet No. 339, 2014). Smoking is estimated to cause about 71% of lung cancer, 42% of chronic respiratory disease and nearly 10% of cardiovascular disease. The proportion of all death attributed to tobacco in the world is from 3% in Africa to 16% in Europe and Americas (WHO global report: mortality attributable to tobacco, 2012). It is strongly connected with smoking prevalence which is lowest in Africa – 15% and highest is Europe – 28% (WHO report on the global tobacco epidemic, 2013). The highest incidence of smoking among men is in lower-middle-income countries; for total population, smoking prevalence is highest among upper-middle-income countries.

The most important health problems connected with smoking are: lung cancer, heart diseases, and tuberculosis. But there are some more side effects like: psoriasis, cataracts, wrinkling, hearing loss, tooth decay, osteoporosis, deformed sperm, discolored fingers, and Buerger's disease. Also other types of cancers are connected with smoking, including nasal and para-nasal cavity cancer, cancer of the oral cavity, nasopharynx cancer; oro and hypopharynx, larynx, esophagus, stomach, pancreas and kidney cancer (Monograph on TB and tobacco control, 2007; Taha, 2012; The Health Consequences of Smoking, 2014; The smoker's body, 2004;).

There are great differences in the incidence of smoking between countries in the European Union. Southern countries see the greatest proportion of smokers, specifically Greece (40% smokers), Bulgaria (38%), Hungary (38%), Turkey (37%) and the Republic of Macedonia (37%). Northern countries have the lowest proportion of smokers: Sweden (16%) and Finland (21%). Socio-demographically, smokers are more likely to be male than female, under 54 years of age and from lower social groups. In terms of occupation, smokers are more likely to be unemployed, manual workers or self-employed (Tobacco; Special Eurobarometer 332, 2010).

In Poland the Global Adult Tobacco Survey (GATS) provided the information that in 2010 33.5% of adult men and 21% of adult women smoked tobacco every day. Around 1.1million Poles smoked occasionally (about 3.3% in both genders). Overall, 30.3% of Poles are current (daily or occasional) smokers. According to OECD Health Data (2012), prevalence of smoking decreased by 14% in Poland during the previous decade.

Some regions of the world like Europe have quite strong smoking policies but there are also countries where the tobacco industry uses plenty of opportunity to persuade people to smoke, e.g. in Africa and Asia. For two decades the WHO has undertaken many initiatives aiming to protect the global population against smoking and the resulting epidemic of tobacco-related diseases. In 2003 the WHO proposed the Framework Convention on Tobacco Control (WHO Framework Convention on Tobacco Control, 2003) which was signed by 168 countries, including the European Community. It indicated the assumptions of the anti-smoking policy which the signatories undertook to implement: price and tax measures to reduce the demand for tobacco, and non-price measures to reduce the demand for tobacco, namely:

– Protection from exposure to tobacco smoke;
– Regulation of the contents of tobacco products;
– Regulation of tobacco product disclosures;
– Packaging and labeling of tobacco products;
– Education, communication, training and public awareness;
– Tobacco advertising, promotion and sponsorship; and,
– Demand reduction measures concerning tobacco dependence and cessation.

The first effects of the implementation of the anti-tobacco policy have been evident already. In Poland, for example, there is a strong decline (-22%) in the prevalence of smoking in eating and drinking establishments, only 5% of respondents noticed smoking people in an eating establishment. In comparison the average percentage for EU is 14%. But there is still much to do, for example to reduce exposure to tobacco at workplace. In Poland only 59% of respondents declare that they are almost never exposed to tobacco, this is a lower percentage compared to the EU average of 72% (Attitudes of Europeans towards tobacco, 2012).

An important role in the preventive actions is played by health professionals. On the one hand, they are professionally prepared in the context of health consequences and treatment of damage from tobacco-related diseases. On the other hand, they simply lack educational competence (including soft skills) related to the consulting role in the process of quitting smoking. Health professionals are not always a good example in this respect, which will be discussed further in this study.

3.4 Alcohol Consumption

The consumption of small amounts of alcohol by adults (up to 12 gram per day) may be beneficial for their bodies as it protects the circulatory system, decreasing the risk of stroke, while alcohol consumption of more than 60 gram per day is associated with an increased relative risk (Reynolds, Lewis, Nolen, Kinney, Sathya, & He, 2003; Ronksley, Brien, Turner, Mukamal, Ghali, & William, 2011). Excessive alcohol consumption is related to an increased risk of such chronic diseases as mouth and oropharyngeal cancers, esophageal cancer, liver cancer, breast cancer, epilepsy, and liver cirrhosis (Rehm, 2003). In the meta-analysis of Corrao, Bagnardi, Zambon and La Vecchia (2004), direct trends in risk were observed for cancers of the oral cavity and pharynx, esophagus, and larynx. Direct relations were also observed for cancers of the colon, rectum, and liver, as well as for breast cancer. Among non-neoplastic conditions, strong direct trends in risk were derived for hypertension, liver cirrhosis, chronic pancreatitis, and injuries and violence (Corrao, Bagnardi, Zambon, & La Vecchia, 2004). Alcohol consumption is associated with neuropsychiatric conditions, like depression or anxiety (Boden & Fergusson, 2011). Harmful use of alcohol weakens the immune system thus enabling development of pneumonia and tuberculosis (Lönnroth, Williams, Stadlin, Jaramillo, & Dye, 2008).

Excessive alcohol consumption is also a significant social problem which not only affects the person abusing alcohol, but also their family, living and working environment, as well as local community and the state. In 2004 the net effects of alcohol consumption on health were detrimental, with an estimated 3.8% of all global deaths and 4.6% of global disability-adjusted life-years attributable to alcohol. In 2012, 5.9% of all global deaths were attributable to alcohol – 7.6% for men, 4.0% for women (Global status report on alcohol and health, 2014). Disease burden is closely related to average volume of alcohol consumption, and, for every unit of exposure, is strongest in poor people and in those who are marginalized from the society. The costs associated with alcohol amount to more than 1% of the gross national product in high-income and middle-income countries, with the costs of social harm constituting a major proportion in addition to health costs (Rehm, 2009).

Due to an equivocal, non-linear link between alcohol and health which is both potentially preventive and definitely harmful, health recommendations in this respect gain particular importance. Another difficulty is related to specifying a standard alcohol dose in the form of one standard drink. Due to historical and geographic determinants, it turns out that one drink is different in different places, for example it amounts to 8 grams of pure alcohol in Ireland and UK, or 19.75 grams in Japan (International drinking guidelines, 2003). Calculations of risk, conducted at a range of alcohol concentrations, take into consideration evidence about the impact of alcohol consumption on overall health and on a number of specific conditions, derived from mortality and morbidity data. While for some individuals no "safe" level of drinking may exist (Dufour, 1999), "safe" or "low risk", "moderate" drinking limits and health recommendations are indicated. For example, physiological differences and different ability to metabolize alcohol between men and women result in differences in recommendations for these groups.

According to the Dietary Guidelines For Americans (2010) moderate consumption of alcohol is defined as up to 1 drink per day (14 g/day) for women and up to 2 drinks per day (28 g/day) for men. Heavy or high-risk drinking is the consumption of more than 3 drinks on any day or more than 7 per week for women and more than 4 drinks on any day or more than 14 per week for men. Binge drinking is the consumption within 2 hours of 4 or more drinks for women and 5 or more drinks for men. The World Health organization promotes the use of the AUDIT instrument (The Alcohol Use Disorders Identification Test), which allows for determining the risk level zones and indicates potential ways of action in primary care. The recommendation for "low-risk" drinking level set in the Guide to Low-Risk Drinking and used in the WHO study on brief interventions is no more than 20 grams of alcohol per day, 5 days a week (recommending at least 2 non-drinking days), and a standard drink equivalent is 10 grams of alcohol (Babor, Higgins-Biddle, Saunders, & Monteiro, 2001). For example: 100 ml glass wine at 12% alc. vol., 30ml nip of high strength spirit at 40% alc. vol., but 285 ml of full strength beer at 4.8% alc. vol. or 60 ml of fortified wine at 20% alc. vol. However recommendations for "low risk" alcohol consumption may be modified to correspond to theAustralian Government webpage: Standard drinks guide national policy and/or local circumstances. Different limits for males, females, and the elderly may be cited (Babor & Higgins-Biddle, 2001).

Alcohol consumption is one of the more important challenges of the EU health policy and it is considered to be a substantial problem in the WHO European Region (Lim et al., 2012), where the highest consumption levels continue to be found in the developed world. In 2010 total alcohol per capita consumption worldwide was

6.2 litres of pure alcohol and 10.9 in Europe (Global status report on alcohol and health, 2014). In the EU in 2004, alcohol was responsible for 1 in 7 male deaths and 1 in 13 female deaths in the group aged 15-64 years (Shield, Kehoe, Gmel, Rehm, & Rehm 2012).

Recent analyses confirm the falling trend in alcohol consumption in some regions of Europe, which is related to lower mortality rate due to alcohol related diseases. However, it is still high, in particular in central and eastern Europe, where a rising trend in alcohol consumption is noted (Anderson & Baumberg, 2006). In Poland alcohol consumption has stabilized in the last decade. Consumption of recorded alcohol increased, while consumption of unrecorded alcohol decreased. In 2010 alcohol consumption per capita (15+) was higher than in the EU – 12.5 litres of pure alcohol (Global status report on alcohol and health, 2014).

3.5 Summary

There are not many specifically dedicated health behaviour standards for health professionals. The well-known standards are those prepared by The Royal College of Physicians and Surgeons of Canada (Puddester et al., 2009). The Canadian physicians are also renowned as having good lifestyles, better than average for the population. However, there is still work to be done on improving standards, because this special professional community needs to deal with very high, not ordinary standards. These individuals have to be the role models for their patients, and they have to be healthy to be able to heal their patients.

4 Health behaviour and its determinants

4.1 Study design

Health behaviours are some of the most essential determinants of our health. This commonly known and accepted statement does not always translate into more health-promoting lifestyles of people. Persons having jobs related to health care or health education are particularly open to being judged by the rest of the society. They include, for example, physicians, nurses and physiotherapists. We can observe a possible opportunity for using the opinion-forming potential of the aforementioned circles and their role in encouraging health behaviours more beneficial to health in patients (clients). One of the basic conditions for the effectiveness of activities taken up by health workers to bring health-promoting lifestyles into focus is their personal example in this regard as well as coherence between educational message and their own behaviour.

To date, the literature in Poland has hardly addressed the issue of preparation of health-promoting activities within medical circles at an individual professional-patient level, especially from the perspective of analysing their own health related behaviours. Until now, more focus has been on the issues of health of medical workers related to professional stress, burning out or occupational diseases.

Somehow, it is assumed that biomedical studies alone will provide future professionals with expertise required for protection and promotion of both their own health and that of their patients. Consequently, it is expected that medical staff will therefore set an example for patients in this sphere of life. This is reflected in the underestimation of the process of education of medical personnel in terms of their pedagogical preparation to provide health education or in the development of so-called soft (social) skills that are so important for good professional-patient relations.

The aim of the present study is to determine the level of implementation and co-occurrence (coherence) of selected health behaviours among present and future medical personnel and to explore differences in their subjective and social determinants. The theoretical background for the proposed subject presentation is based on a holistic health model and in particular a socio-ecological approach (Capra 1982). The proposed research model (Fig. 4.1 and 4.2) was based on the TTI model and the assumptions for the study included the use of elements of the Bandura's Social Cognitive Theory (Bandura, 1986) and Rotter's expectancy-reinforcement model (Rotter, 1966), transposed to the field of health (Laverson, 1974).

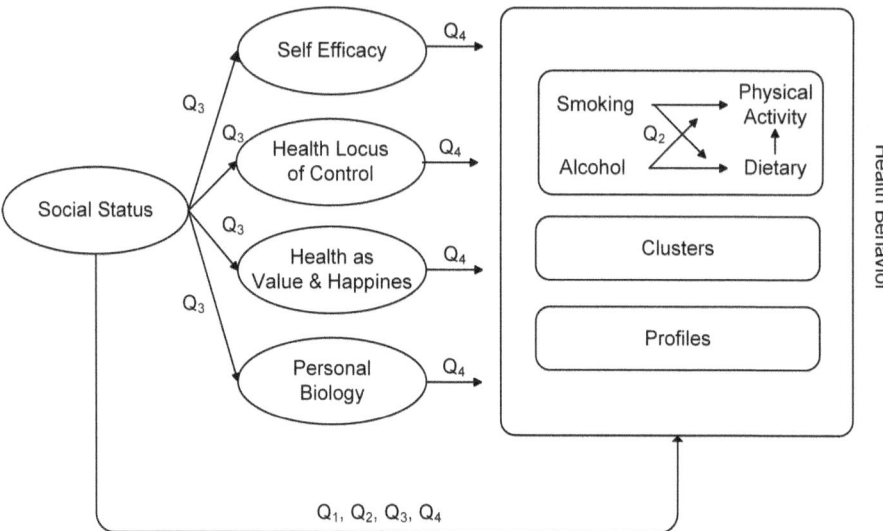

Figure 4.1 Proposed research model

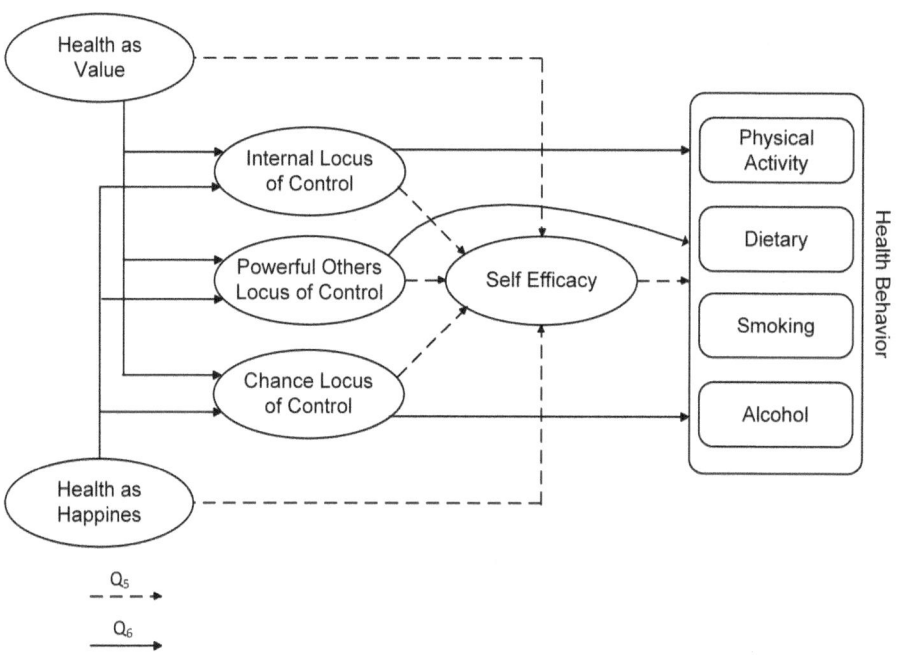

Figure 4.2 Proposed research model – mediating models (Q5, Q6)

Based on a review of the literature on the subject, the following research questions were formulated:

Q 1. What is the level of health behaviour by present and future medical personnel?

Q 2. Is there a significant co-occurrence of the examined health behaviours (both beneficial and adverse) revealed in the groups of respondents participating in the study? Is it possible to define clusters of health behaviours typical of the selected social and professional groups?

Q 3. Do the groups of present and future medical professionals significantly differ in terms of the selected subject variables (self-rated health, health valuation, perceived health locus of control, self-efficacy) in respect of the selected health behaviours and biological indices (BMI, WHR, incidence of lifestyle diseases)?

Q 4. Which variables (subject, biological, social) correlate with health behaviour, health behaviour clusters and health profiles of both present and future medical personnel?

Q 5. Does self-efficacy play a mediator role in the relationship between health valuation and health behaviour as well as between health locus of control and health behaviour?

Q 6. Does health locus of control play a mediator role in the relationship between health valuation and health behaviour?

Table 4.1 presents the variables subject to analysis in the study together with indexes for their assessment and research tools used.

Table 4.1 Variables and their operationalization

Variables	Indicators	Tools
Health Behaviour		
Physical Activity	level of PA (low, medium, high) METs	The International Physical Activity Questionnaire (IPAQ short version)
Nutrition	Nutrition Index 12 (points:12-36) Nutrition Index 3 (points:3-9) level: low, medium, high	author's questionnaire *Me and My Health*
Smoking	categories: current, ex-, never smoking	author's questionnaire *Me and My Health*
Alcohol Consumption	categories: abstinent, moderate, high, binge	author's questionnaire *Me and My Health*
Health Behaviour Profiles	categories: destructive, ambivalent, passive, average, beneficial	author's questionnaire *Me and My Health*
Self-rated Health (SRH)	categories: very good, good, moderate, bad, very bad	World Health Survey, WHO (2002)

continued**Table 4.1** Variables and their operationalization

Variables	Indicators	Tools
Health-Specific Self-Efficacy		
Physical Exercise Self-Efficacy	points (5-20) level: low, medium, high	Physical Exercise Self-Efficacy Scale (Schwarzer & Renner, 2000a)
Nutrition Self-Efficacy	points (5-20) level: low, medium, high	Nutrition Self-Efficacy Scale (Schwarzer & Renner, 2000a)
Smoking Self-Efficacy	points (9-36) level: low, medium, high	Smoking Self-Efficacy Questionnaire (Velicer et.al., 1990)
Alcohol Resistance Self-Efficacy	points (3-15) level: low, medium, high	Alcohol Resistance Self-Efficacy Scale (Schwarzer & Renner, 2000a)
Health as a personal value	range: from 0 (not chosen) to 5 (the most important)	List of Personal Value (LPV) (Juczyński, 2001)
Health as a happiness symbol	range: from 0 (not chosen) to 5 (the most important)	List of Personal Value (LPV) (Juczyński, 2001)
Health Locus of Control	Internal: points (6-36), level: low, high Powerful Others: points (6-36), level: low, high Chance: points (6-36), level: low, high	Multidimensional Health Locus of Control Scale (MHCL) (Wallston et. al., 1978; Juczyński, 2001)
Socio-demographic status	stage of education: student, professional occupation: physician, nurse, physiotherapist, medical student, physiotherapy student age (years) gender marital status (categories: single, married, divorced, widow/er) material status (categories: excellent, good, average, poor)	demographic survey
Biological Heath Indicator	BMI: value, categories Waist circumference Waist-hip Ratio chronic diseases	author's questionnaire *Me and My Health*

The following groups of independent variables were taken into consideration in the study during statistical analyses:
1. Subject variables (Self-rated Health (SRH), Health-Specific Self-Efficacy, Health as a personal value, Health as a happiness symbol, Health Locus of Control)
2. Social variables – career stage (student – major in biomedical studies, professional – graduate of biomedical studies), occupation (medical student, physiotherapy student, physician, nurse, physiotherapist)

3. Biological variables (BMI, Waist circumference, Waist-hip Ratio, chronic diseases).

Dependent variables include health behaviours of both future and current medical personnel presented in two ways: as individual behaviours (physical activity, nutrition, smoking, alcohol consumption) or as Health Behaviour Profiles the construction of which is discussed in the description of research tools.

The following section outlines the research tools used.

To assess **health-specific self-efficacy** we used free questionnaires developed by Schwarzer and Renner (2000a): **The Nutrition Self-Efficacy Scale, The Physical Exercise Self-Efficacy Scale, The Alcohol Resistance Self-Efficacy Scale,** and the **Smoking Self-Efficacy Questionnaire** developed by Velicer and others (1990). The following responses were proposed for all statements included in the questionnaires and regarding health-related self-efficacy: very uncertain (1 point), rather uncertain (2 points), rather certain (3 points) and very certain (4 points). Next, the total value for each scale was determined and the scores obtained for the surveyed population were converted to standard ten scores (stens) where the score below 5 sten scores was considered as "low level", from 5 to 6 inclusive as medium level and from 7 upwards as "high level".

The Nutrition Self-Efficacy Scale includes five statements regarding the certainty of respondents as to their ability to deal with barriers that may hinder the preparation of healthy foods. The Physical Exercise Self-Efficacy Scale includes also five statements referring to the potential obstacles to carrying out exercises by respondents. The Alcohol Resistance Self-Efficacy Scale contains three potential situations that may affect the respondents' ability to control themselves. The Smoking Self-Efficacy Questionnaire includes nine potential situations in which the confidence of respondents in their ability to refrain from smoking is verified.

In accordance with the questionnaire adaptation procedure, the self-efficacy questionnaires were translated into Polish by two independent translators (English Philology graduates) and verified by 3 competent judges (PhDs in Physical Culture Sciences, two with specialisation in Health Education). Tests verifying the questionnaire reliability were conducted among 116 adults and Cronbach's alpha for individual scales was between 0.66 and 0.78.

To assess the **health locus of control** we used the **Multidimensional Health Locus of Control Scale** (Wallston, 1978; Juczyński, 2001). The Multidimensional Health Locus of Control Scale (MHLC) consists of 18 statements for which a Likert-scale of summated ratings was used and numerical values were assigned to each of the six possible responses. For statements in which a favorable response was desired, a "strongly agree" was assigned a numerical value of 6 and a "strongly disagree" a numerical value of 1. According to the authors' proposal, it allows the classification of results using the median as a point of division between high and low results in each of the health control dimensions: **Internal** Health Locus of Control (IHLC),

Powerful Others Health Locus of Control (PHLC), and **Chance** Health Locus of Control (CHLC). The IHLC scale assesses individuals' ability to control their health. The PHLC scale tests the beliefs that powerful others, such as doctors, nurses, friends, and family, determine one's health. The CHLC construct assesses the beliefs that health or illness was determined by fate, luck, or chance. In the study the A version of the questionnaire was used for which the Polish adaptation as well as validity and reliability assessments were made by Juczyński (2001).

The **List of Personal Values (LPV)** (Juczyński, 2001) allows respondents to assess health as a value in the context of other values. The questionnaire consists of two parts. In the first one each respondent chooses 5 (out of 9) *symbols of happiness* (many friends, satisfying family life, doing favorite job, success in education, work, good health, being needed by others, good financial situation, life full of adventure, fame and popularity) and ranks (classifies) them from the most important one (5 points) to the least important one (1 point). A similar procedure is followed in the second part where the respondent chooses 5 (out of 10) *personal values* (love and friendship, good health and physical fitness, sense of humor, intelligence, wisdom, courage, joy, kindness, good looks, wealth) and then ranks them. In the designed studies the classification (ranking) made by respondents will be used for determining correlations with the demonstrated health behaviours.

Self-rated Health (SRH). In accordance with the guidelines of the World Health Organization (World Health Survey, 2002) the following question was used for the subjective health assessment: "In general, how would you rate your health today?". The respondents provided answers using a scale of five: "very good, good, moderate, bad, very bad".

The International Physical Activity Questionnaire (IPAQ short version) (Biernat & Stupnicki, 2005, Craig et al., 2003) was used to assess the respondents' physical activity. Metabolic Equivalent values (METs) per week were calculated for individuals and the respondents were divided into three categories of PA (low, moderate, high). The questionnaire includes 7 questions regarding: intensive and moderate physical efforts made in the most recent month as well as movement activity (walking) and time spent sitting.

The author's questionnaire *Me and My Health* was used to assess **nutrition, alcohol consumption** and **smoking status**. It also contains questions about **anthropometric dimensions** (weight, height, waist and hip circumference), lifestyle diseases and **socio-demographic status**.

The nutrition status was calculated as a mean of answers to 12 questions. The questions were constructed in accordance with the guidelines of the National Food and Nutrition Institute (Principles of Proper Nutrition, 2009) and recommendations included in the Golden Charter of Proper Nutrition (1997). This document constitutes a consensus reached by numerous organizations dealing with the promotion of healthy nutrition within the scope of nutritional recommendations for healthy adults. The analysis was also based on the guidelines included in the so-called Healthy Eating

Pyramid (2009), still constituting one of the socially most recognizable symbols of nutritional recommendations, despite the criticism of its assumptions.

The questionnaire contained questions regarding: frequency of meals (including in particular breakfasts) and frequency of consumption of certain products: whole grain products, vegetables, fruits, dairy, legumes, fish, white meat, red meat, vegetable oil, water (on a 5-point scale from "every day" to "never").

In order to to analyse respondents' nutrition behaviours as one component (variable) and to also take all the analysed eating habits into consideration a summary index was proposed, allowing us to determine the level of adoption of the studied nutrition behaviours by the respondents – Nutrition Index. Having given consideration to health guidelines, following consultation with nutrition specialists at the Poznań University of Life Sciences, individual behaviours were classified as adverse, moderately beneficial or beneficial to health by assigning the score of 1, 2 and 3 to them, respectively. As a result, each respondent could get the score between 12 and 26 in respect of the nutrition index, taking all 12 studied nutrition behaviours into consideration (Nutrition Index 12, NI12). Next, the scores obtained for the surveyed population were converted to standard ten scores, where the score below 5 sten scores was considered as "low level", from 5 to 6 inclusive as "medium level" and from 7 upwards as "high level". Given the fact that the consumed complex carbohydrates, vegetables and fruits are considered to be particularly important diet elements in terms of health, also Nutrition Index 3 (NI3), taking these behaviours into consideration, was proposed. The score that could be achieved in respect of NI3 ranged from 3 to 9. It was found that in order to be considered beneficial to health the NI3 index must contain maximum one of the studied behaviours at the moderate level whereas the others must be definitely beneficial. It gives a score of 8 or 9 for "high level", 7 for "medium level" and 6 or below for "low level".

Smoking status was evaluated in three categories: as currently smoking, ex-smoking or non-smoking respondents. It was also evaluated if the respondents are passive smokers.

The assessment of behaviours related to **alcohol consumption** was made on the basis of both frequency and quantity of consumed alcohol portions (so-called standard drinks). A standard drink is considered to contain 10 g of pure alcohol that can be found, for example, in 1 glass of wine (100 ml), 1 shot of vodka (25 ml) or 1 glass of beer (250 ml). 4 patterns of alcohol consumption were distinguished on that basis (Dietary Guidelines for Americans, 2010; CDC. Fact Sheets – Preventing Excessive Alcohol Use, n.d.): an abstinent is a person who declares that he/she does not drink alcohol, moderate alcohol consumption is defined as up to 1 drink per day for women and up to 2 drinks per day for men, high-risk drinking is the consumption of more than 7 drinks per week for women and more than 14 per week for men, binge drinking is the consumption of 4 or more drinks for women and 5 or more drinks for men per day.

The first version of the *Me and My Health* questionnaire was verified and used during the studies conducted in 1997, serving as a part of preparations for doctoral dissertation of the author of the project entitled: *Determinants of pro-health activities in the workplace with the allocation of a place for physical activity.* For the purposes of the designed study it was modified and extended to include the need for classification of the behaviours subject to analysis. The questionnaire reliability was verified in a study conducted on 189 students of the University School of Physical Education in Poznań. The study was conducted using a test-retest method at an interval of 3 weeks and the correlation coefficient for individual questions ranged between 0.67 and 0.88.

Health Behaviour Profiles. The paper proposes an original approach to the comprehensive analysis of health behaviours. The behaviours subject to study were divided into two groups: (1) health-enhancing behaviours (physical activity, nutrition beneficial to health), i.e. the behaviours in which the respondents' activities prove to be beneficial to their health and (2) health-compromising behaviours (smoking, excessive consumption of alcohol), i.e. the behaviours in which the respondents' activities prove to be adverse to their health. Each of the distinguished groups included 2 health behaviours classified on a 3-point scale: adverse (low PA, low NI12, current smoker, binge or heavy alcohol consumption), moderate (moderate PA, moderate NI12, ex-smoker, moderate alcohol consumption), beneficial (high PA, high NI12, never smoker, abstinent). Next, the co-occurrence was calculated for the health-enhancing behaviours and for the health-compromising behaviours (-,+,++; see legend in Tab. 4.2), respectively, whereas the last stage included the taxonomization of co-occurrence of all the four behaviours. Based on such division of the analysed health behaviour, it is possible to distinguish various types of human activity related to one's health (Health Behaviour Profiles), as illustrated in Table 4.2.

Table 4.2 Matrix for Health Behaviour Profiles

Taxonomy of activity related to health		Health-enhancing behaviours		
		-	+	++
Health-compromising behaviours	++		*Ambivalent*	
	+	*Destructive*	*Average*	
	-	*Passive*	*Beneficial*	

Legend: (-) – no occurrence of behaviours, activity; (+) – moderate intensity of behaviour, activity occurrence; (++) – intensive occurrence of behaviours, activity

A *destructive* Health Behaviour Profile was found to be the one in which there are no health-enhancing behaviours or there is a moderate or intensive occurrence of health-compromising behaviours. It may involve the co-occurrence of: low physical activity, adverse diet, binge or heavy alcohol consumption and ex-smoking or smoking status. A *passive* Health Behaviour Profile was found to be the one in which there are no health-enhancing behaviours and no health-compromising behaviours. It may involve the co-occurrence of: low physical activity, adverse diet, being an abstinent and never smoking status. An *ambivalent* Health Behaviour Profile was found to be the one in which on the one hand there are health-enhancing behaviours but on the other hand the occurrence of health-compromising behaviours is intensive. It may involve the co-occurrence of: moderate or high physical activity, beneficial diet, binge or heavy alcohol consumption and ex-smoking or smoking status. An *average* Health Behaviour Profile was found to be the one in which on the one hand there are health-enhancing behaviours but on the other hand the occurrence of health-compromising behaviours is moderately intensive. It may involve the co-occurrence of: moderate or high physical activity, beneficial diet, binge or heavy alcohol consumption and never smoking status. A *beneficial* Health Behaviour Profile was found to be the one in which on the one hand there are health-enhancing behaviours and on the other hand there are no health-compromising behaviours. It may involve the co-occurrence of: moderate or high physical activity, beneficial diet, being an abstinent and never smoking status.

Biological variables. The respondents were asked to independently assess the following parameters: weight and height, allowing calculation of the **Body Mass Index** (BMI). It is defined as the weight in kilograms divided by the square of the height in meters (kg/m^2). Due to the discussion of experts on the BMI classification and the need for a revision of the cut-off point of 25 kg/m^2 defining overweight in the current WHO classification, it was decided to take also an additional cut-off point of 23 kg/m^2 into account in the analysis. BMI classification according to the WHO recommendations (1995, 2000, 2004) applied in the paper:

– underweight <18.50
– normal range I 18.50-22.99 (additional cut-off point)
– normal range II 23.00-24.99
– overweight ≥25.00
– obese ≥30.

The respondents were also asked to measure **waist and hip circumferences**. The results obtained were treated rather as a rough guide since they were not obtained from measures professionally taken by trained interviewers. However, it should be noted that the professional groups being studied are properly instructed in taking such measures and it may be assumed that a proportion of false readings would be lower than for the general population. On that basis a **Waist-Hip Ratio** was calculated whereas the waist circumference was also used for determining the risk of metabolic complications. Based on these two WHO recommendations (Waist Circumference and Waist–Hip Ratio, 2011), it was found that the increased risk occurred in the case of waist circumference >94 cm for men and >80 cm women; substantially increased risk was present in the case of individuals with waist circumferences >102 cm for men and >88 cm for women. For waist waist-hip ratio the values ≥0.90 for men and ≥0.85 for women were found resulting in the increased risk of metabolic complications. The respondents were also asked about the presence of **chronic diseases**, such as: hypertension, varicose veins, obesity, atherosclerosis, peptic ulcer disease, diabetes, allergies, asthma, depression or cardiovascular disease.

4.1.1 Survey Process and Study Participants

In the study we used the diagnostic survey employing a Snowball Sampling method (Atkinson & Flint, 2001). We used this method especially for the investigation of a group of health professionals because it is very difficult to convince them to take part in such a survey. An anonymous questionnaire survey was conducted. It took around 20-30 minutes to complete. The participation in the survey was voluntary and this strategy helped to obtain responses. The study participants included health professionals from randomly chosen hospitals, medical clinics and rehabilitation clinics in Poznań and Wielkopolska Provinces in Poland. The survey was also conducted among physiotherapy students at the University School of Physical Education in Poznań and among medical students at the Poznań University of Medical Sciences. The survey among students was conducted during educational classes (usually at the end of the lecture) and the participation was voluntary so any student unwilling to participate had an option to leave the lecture hall. The survey was conducted in 2011 and 2012.

The study gathered data from 777 individuals, including 428 medical and physiotherapy students and 349 medical professionals. The stratification of the participants is presented in Table 4.3.

Table 4.3 Description of the study samples

		All	students		professionals		
			medical	physiotherapy	physicians	nurses	physiotherapists
n (%)		777	223 (28.7)	205 (26.4)	111 (14.3)	114 (14.7)	124 (15.9)
age	M ± SD	29.4±12.0	21.4±1.7	20.6±1.2	41.1±11.3	44.4±8.3	33.8±11.2
gender n (%)	♀	580 (74.6)	165 (74.0)	146 (71.2)	83 (74.8)	105 (92.1)	81 (65.3)
	♂	197 (25.4)	58 (26.0)	59 (28.8)	28 (25.2)	9 (7.9)	43 (34.7)
marital status n (%)	single	500 (64.4)	206 (92.4)	202 (98.0)	20 (18.0)	15 (13.2)	57 (46.0)
	married	243 (31.3)	9 (4.0)	0 (0.0)	88 (79.3)	94 (82.5)	52 (42.0)
	divorced	14 (1.8)	0 (0.0)	0 (0.0)	1 (0.9)	0 (0.0)	13 (10.5)
	widow/er	6 (0.8)	0 (0.0)	0 (0.0)	2 (1.8)	3 (2.6)	1 (0.8)
material status n (%)	excellent	66 (8.5)	23 (10.3)	18 (8.8)	20 (18.0)	2 (1.8)	3 (2.4)
	good	485 (62.4)	138 (61.9)	113 (55.1)	77 (69.4)	83 (72.8)	74 (59.7)
	average	217 (28.0)	58 (26.0)	69 (33.7)	14 (12.6)	29 (25.4)	47 (37.9))
	poor	3 (0.4)	0 (0.0)	3 (1.5)	0 (0.0)	0 (0.0)	0 (0.0)

Note: numbers may not add to total due to missing data

4.1.2 Statistical Analysis

The study was based on a correlation-regression model meaning that it is only possible to draw conclusions regarding correlations between variables rather than making cause-effect interpretations. A mediation analysis was also used in order to explicate relationships between independent and dependent variables through analysing the impact of intermediate variables. However, in this case there is no strict control over variables like in an experimental model and that's why, caution was exercised in their interpretation.

In the first stage of the analysis the respondents were characterized within the scope of the examined variables and differences were sought between them. Depending on the tool and the variable, some descriptive statistics were used, including the arithmetic mean, standard deviation, and percentages for individual categories. In order to compare the groups parametric tests were used for continuous variables while comparing two groups – Student's t-distribution together with Hedges's g effect size index for which the following effect size classification was adopted: 0.2 – small effect size, 0.5 – medium effect size, 0.8 – large effect size. In comparisons of more groups a one-way analysis of variance (ANOVA) was used for which next post hoc Tukey test and eta squared effect size were calculated for which the following effect size classification was adopted: 0.01 – small effect size, 0.06 – medium effect size, 0.14 – large effect size. For ranked variables non-parametric tests were used: for the comparison of two groups – the Mann-Whitney U test with the Glass's rank biserial correlation coefficient (r_g) for which the following effect size classification was adopted: 0.2 – small effect size, 0.5 – medium effect size, 0.8 – large effect size. In comparisons of more groups the Kruskal-Wallis test was used for which next post hoc tests for comparisons between the groups as well as Epsilon-squared effect size were calculated for which the following effect size classification was adopted: 0.1 – small effect size, 0.3 – medium effect size, 0.5 – large effect size. In comparisons of categorical variables the chi-square test was used for which next the Cramer's V effect size was calculated for which the following effect size classification was adopted: 0.1 – small effect size, 0.3 – medium effect size, 0.5 – large effect size. The two-way ANOVA was also used in order to determine relationships and interaction between the successively selected health behaviours and group/or career stage effect on the level of the other health behaviour. We set the level of significance a priori at p< .05 (Cohen, 1988; King & Minium, 2009).

In the next stage of the study the analysis of clusters was employed in order to determine the co-occurrence of health behaviours. It is a tool designed to reveal natural groupings (clusters) within a data set that would otherwise not be apparent. A two-step cluster analysis procedure was employed which allowed us to analyse both qualitative and quantitative variables at the same time (Norusis, 2006). The variables on the basis of which clusters were identified included four lifestyle risk factors: physical activity, nutrition, smoking and alcohol consumption. The following indicators of behaviours were chosen: two levels of physical activity: low or moderate and high; sum of points for NI12 for nutrition; three levels for smoking: current smoking, ex-smoking, never smoking; two levels for alcohol consumption: moderate and heavy or binge drinking. In order to minimize the effect of the order of observations in the sample on the clustering results the set was sorted by randomly generated numbers. The measure of distance between clusters was based on a log-likelihood ratio whereas the Schwarz's Bayesian Information Criterion was used as a clustering criterion. The analyses were run in the SPSS 21.0 programme.

The subsequent stage of the analysis involved the search for relationships between the indicated determinants of health behaviours and the degree of adoption of given health behaviours. To accomplish that purpose, a logistic regression was employed. For that purpose, the dependent variables were classified as dichotomous variables and the conversion details were described next to the study results. The analyses were run in the Statistica 10 programme.

The last stage of the analysis involved the use of mediation analysis. The mediation analysis is one of the most popular and standard procedures employed in social sciences in order to explicate relationships between independent and dependent variables based on the search for mediators (Hayes, 2009, 2013; MacKinnon, Fairchild, & Fritz, 2007; Rucker, Preacher, Tormala, & Petty, 2011). In order to prove that a given variable is a mediating factor bringing us closer to the explanation of a relationship between the independent variable and the dependent variable it is necessary to take a few steps. In the classic approach it involves (Baron & Kenny, 1986): (1) demonstrating a correlation between the independent and dependent variables – path "c" (Fig. 4.3); (2) demonstrating that the independent variable correlates with the intervening variable – path "a" (Fig. 4.3) and (3) demonstrating that the intervening variable correlates with the dependent variable, even taking the independent variable in the model into consideration – path "b" (Fig. 4.3). It is expected that the original relationship between the independent variable and the dependent one (path coefficient "c" – total effect) will decrease to an insignificant value at the adopted level of significance (coefficient "c'" – direct effect). In the classic mediation approach such decrease proves the complete mediation. However, in practice a partial decrease of the contribution of the independent variable to the dependent one is often observed, proving the partial mediation which allows the assumption that there are other mechanisms regulating the relationship between the variables.

Currently, most scientific research methodologists find it of key importance for mediation to demonstrate a relationship between the independent variable and the dependent variable – path coefficient "a" and a relationship between the intervening variable and the dependent variable – path coefficient "b" (Fig. 4.1). An analysis of statistical significance and indirect effect size – "a" x "b" (Fig. 4.1) is conducted without placing any emphasis on demonstrating a statistically significant relationship between the independent variable and the dependent variable (Hayes, 2009; Rucker et al., 2011; Zhao, Lynch, & Chen, 2010). Consequently, it is believed that the mediation hypothesis should be considered confirmed when a statistically

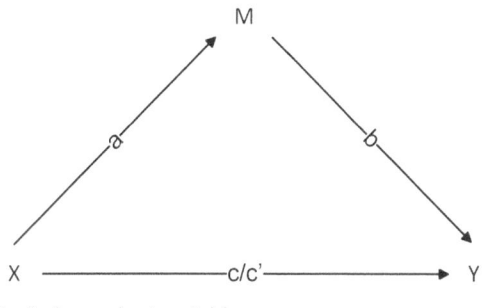

X – independent variable
M – mediator
Y – dependent variable

Figure 4.3 Diagram of relationships in the classic mediation analysis (Baron & Kenny, 1986)

significant, essentially justified indirect effect is obtained (Hayes, 2009, 2013; Rucker et al., 2011; Zhao et al., 2010). Therefore, such interpretation was adopted in this paper for the mediation analysis. The null hypothesis of indirect effect was tested with the use of a non-parametric bootstraping procedure recommended by Preacher and Hayes (2008). The effect size for path "a" of the mediation model is indicated by the values of correlation coefficients adequate to the usual values for correlation coefficients proposed by Cohen (1988) for using in social science studies where the correlation coefficient of 0.1 represents a small effect size, 0.30 – a medium effect size and 0.50 – a large effect size. The coefficient of path "b" (beta weight β) indicates how much the value of the dependent value will change if the value of the mediator changes by one standard deviation, with the independent variable being controlled. In the models calculated in this paper the standardized coefficients are close to the coefficients of partial correlation; therefore, the assessment of path "b" may be made based on the interpretation of correlation effect sizes: product indirect effect value of 0.01 represents a small effect size, 0.09 – a medium effect size and 0.25 – a large effect size (Shrout & Bolger, 2002). The mediation analysis was conducted with the use of the SPSS macro recommended by Preacher and Hayes (2009, 2013).

4.2 Health behaviour of medical and physiotherapy students and professionals

The variables being examined in this study include four basic health behaviours of future and present medical personnel: physical activity, nutrition, smoking and alcohol consumption. These are the most important behaviours related to health which are also the most common risk factors for lifestyle diseases. Usually, the epidemiological structure of the occurrence of individual behaviours is subject to analysis. However, a special concern may be raised by the accumulation of adverse behaviours in particular social groups. Therefore, the aim of this part of the study is to analyse the level of the four main health behaviours (physical activity, nutrition, smoking, alcohol consumption) and the patterns of their co-occurrence among medical students and professionals. The study will also result in distinguishing the so-called "weakest links" in the lifestyle of the respondents, i.e. behaviours adverse to health frequently occurring in the social groups subject to analysis. We will also attempt to identify differences in the frequency of occurrence of specific Health Behaviour Profiles (*destructive, passive, ambivalent, average, beneficial*) in the social and professional groups subject to analysis.

4.2.1 Physical Activity

Unsurprisingly, both students and graduates of the University School of Physical Education lead the way in physical activity (Tab. 4.4). The level of physical activity of physiotherapy students and physiotherapists is significantly higher than that of nurses (p<.0001 and p<.0001, respectively) and physicians (p=.0010 and p=.0412, respectively). The nurses participating in the study are characterized by particularly low physical activity that is also significantly lower than physical activity of medical students (p=.0012). The social and professional diversification of the respondents (in this case affiliation to one of the following groups studied: physiotherapy students, medical students, physiotherapists, physicians, nurses) explains approximately 5% difference in the level of physical activity of respondents (p<.0001). Also, a higher level of physical activity, on average, can be observed in students compared to professionals (p<.0001, Hedges' g=.318). Gender shows no effects.

Table 4.4 Descriptive characteristics and test statistics for differences in respondents' physical activity

PA [a]	All	students			professionals			
		all	medical	physio-therapy	all	physi-cians	nurses	physio-thera-pists
Low n (%)	157 (20.4)	62 (14.5)	36 (16.1)	26 (12.7)	95 (27.9)	29 (26.8)	45 (41.7)	21 (16.9)
Medium n (%)	224 (29.2)	132 (30.8)	80 (35.9)	52 (25.4)	92 (27.1)	37 (34.3)	23 (21.3)	32 (25.8)
High n (%)	387 (50.4)	234 (54.7)	107 (48.0)	127 (61.9)	153 (45.0)	42 (38.9)	40 (37.0)	71 (57.3)

	all groups			students/professionals		
	F	p value	η^2	t	p value	Hedges' g
PA (METs) [b]	10.793	<.0001	.05	4.09	<.0001	.318

[a] - *according to IPAQ score PA measure in METs and divided in 3 categories;*

[b] - *test t or one way ANOVA were used for differences between studied groups; effect size: Hedges's g, eta-squared (η^2)*

As people grow older, their level of physical activity decreases and this fact is clearly reflected in the scores obtained by the respondents. A professional group that is most exposed to health consequences of low physical activity among the respondents is that of nurses. Numerous studies exist documenting the professional difficulties (both physical and mental) of nurses. Often these can also serve as "excuses" or form objective obstacles to following more active lifestyles. Clearly, fatigue associated with professional duties, combined most frequently with low salaries, do not contribute to the implementation of health recommendations in that regard.

Another question is how educationally effective a medical service worker can be, especially in the context of the process of internalising his/her behaviours by patients, in a situation in which every fourth physician and almost every second nurse participating in the study do not meet a minimum health criterion in that regard.

4.2.2 Nutrition

Nutrition is one of the basic determinants of health. It may promote and build health or contribute to the occurrence of diseases, in particular lifestyle diseases (chronic). The professional groups studied have nutrition education included in their training process. All standards concerning best practices related to medical profession contain provisions showing the need for those specialists to implement elements of health education, including nutrition education. It is anticipated that this would be reflected in the implementation of good standards of health behaviour in this field by the professionals themselves.

Nutrition behaviours of the respondents were analysed based on the recommendations set out in the Golden Chart of Proper Nutrition (1997) and the guidelines of the National Food and Nutrition Institute (2009). Those documents constitute a consensus reached by numerous organizations dealing with the promotion of healthy nutrition within the scope of nutritional recommendations for healthy adults. The elements that play a special role in diet-related disease prevention include the consumption of vegetables and fruits as well as whole grain products. Moreover, the analysis focused on the type and frequency of consumption of dairy products, leguminous plants, meat, fish and plant oils, body hydration as well as the regularity and number of meals consumed during a day. The respondents indicated the frequency of consumption of individual products during a week or at rarer intervals. Table 5 presents a percentage of persons implementing health beneficial nutrition recommendations.

The highest percentage of individuals implementing beneficially healthy recommendations includes 80% of respondents who consume white meat (poultry) several times a week. On the one hand, this can be seen as a positive change because poultry is healthier than red meat. On the other hand, this is not necessarily what actually happens since the percentage of persons choosing red meat products

Table 4.5 Percentage (%) of respondents pursuing beneficial dietary patterns.

dietary patterns	All %	students %			professionals %			
		all	medical	physiotherapy	all	physicians	nurses	physiotherapists
vegetables every day	45.3	41.8	52.0	30.5	49.6	55.0	39.5	54.0
fruits every day	39.5	32.2	35.0	29.3	48.4	56.8	46.5	42.7
whole grains every day	49.2	49.3	57.4	40.5	49.0	45.0	36.8	63.7
dairy every day	34.1	31.5	32.7	30.2	37.2	61.3	24.6	27.4
legumes few days in the week	23.8	20.2	20.2	20.2	28.2	33.3	23.3	28.2
white meat few days in the week	79.1	78.2	78,5	78.0	80.2	67,5	90.3	82.3
red meat rarely or never	29.4	31.0	27.3	34.9	27.5	29.7	25.5	27.4
fish few days in the week	46.8	41.7	41.7	41.7	53.1	50.4	58.1	50.8
vegetable oils few days in the week	47.1	52.1	47.1	57.6	40.9	39.6	49.1	34.6
water, vegetable juices every day	56.4	65.6	77.6	52.7	45.3	53.1	34.2	48.4
breakfast always	72.5	69.8	68.5	71.2	75.9	82.7	71.9	73.4
the number of meals >3	69.5	75.0	80.3	69.3	62.6	60.0	63.2	64.5

less frequently is quite low, around 30%. The popularity of poultry is driven not only by health reasons but also by its price and ease of preparation. Particularly alarming are the statistics for everyday consumption of vegetables, fruits and whole grain products. None of the recommendations were implemented by even a half of the total respondents. Nurses and physiotherapy students compare particularly unfavorably in this regard. Only a third of respondents consume milk and dairy products every day. Milk is the subject of much controversy and reports about its harmfulness and excessive consumption have been reported in the Polish media. Half-truths and the lack of factual reporting of the issue may, affect respondents' consumption. Interestingly, physicians compare significantly favorably in this regard with over 60% consuming dairy products every day. Similarly, legumes are included more often in their diet though they still are not popular products among the respondents. Only one in four respondents consume them frequently enough, with slightly more frequent consumption among professionals compared to students. Despite a number of advertising campaigns promoting the consumption of fish and the tradition of abstaining from eating meat on Fridays and replacing it with fish, still maintained by many Polish families, fewer than half of respondents eat fish several times a week (one time at minimum). Plant oils and margarines have become more and more popular and they are used for various purposes in Polish kitchens. Still, most often they are used for frying and that's why their consumption is not recommended on a daily basis, also due to trans fats in hydrogenated margarines. These patterns are followed by almost a half of the respondents. In order to comment on the special role of fats in the respondents' diets it would be necessary to analyse their dietary patterns in greater detail than allowed by the scope of this study. It may only be assumed that oils are used increasingly often and saturated fats are partially supplanted by them in cooking. Neither water nor vegetable and fruit juices are included in the everyday menu of the respondents. It may be assumed that they supplement fluids with other drinks, including sweetened carbonated beverages which, as is well known, are one of the most important factors contributing to overweight and obesity. The proper number of meals per day is declared by almost 70% of respondents, especially students (75%). Clearly, their organization of both work and leisure time during the academic year contributes to getting the proper number of meals better than professional duties of physicians, nurses or physiotherapists (63%). Professionals, however, appreciate more the value (role) of breakfast, with only 24% of them starting their day without this meal. In the group of students it amounts to approx. 30%. The presented degree of implementation of the selected beneficial dietary habits of the current and future medical personnel causes great concern and offers a wide field for education and promotion interventions which, as it turns out, are needed also in the case of health educators.

According to the procedure described in the chapter on research tools, two summary indexes, namely Nutrition Index 12 (NI12) and Nutrition Index 3 (NI3), were distinguished for the evaluation of dietary habits. The first one took all twelve nutrition behaviours (see Tab. 4.5 above) into account and each respondent got a score between 12 and 36; moreover, the NI12 values were converted to standard ten scores and classified as low, medium or high. On the other hand, the other index included three basic health-protective diet elements, i.e. the consumption of complex carbohydrates, vegetables and fruits, and it allowed the classification of behaviours as adverse, moderate and beneficial. The characteristics and differences related to the Nutrition Indexes are presented in Table 4.6.

The obtained results relating to nutrition behaviours (NI12) clearly show that the diet of professionals is better than that of students (p=.0113, Hedges' g=-.185). While analyzing average NI12 scores for individual groups, we can also see significant differences among them (p=.0005, η^2=.03). In this context, physiotherapy students compare particularly unfavorably to physiotherapists (p=.0412) and physicians (p=.0004) whereas nurses compare significantly worse than physicians (p=.0379).

Differences can be observed in the consumption of the three health-essential diet elements (complex carbohydrates, vegetables and fruits) – NI3 – among present and future medical personnel, in favor of the first group (p<.0001, Hedges' g=-.349). The result shows significant differences between groups (p<.0001, η^2=.06) with physiotherapy students demonstrating worse nutrition behaviour than other groups (p<.0001 compared to physiotherapists and physicians, p=.0289 compared to nurses and p=.0018 compared to medical students). On the other hand, physiotherapists compare favorably to nurses (p=.0488), physiotherapy students (p<.0001) and medical students (p=.0229).

Gender differentiates the respondents in terms of the implemented dietary patterns (NI12). Men demonstrate worse nutrition behaviour more often than women (p=.0015, η^2=.01). When analyzing differences in individual social and professional groups we can find them among physiotherapists (p=.0043) and medical students (p=.0004). The analysis focusing only on the three most important health behaviours (the NI3) reveals again that it is women who implement more health-promoting nutrition (p<.0001, η^2=.02). We can also observe better nutrition indices in women than in men among physiotherapists (p=.0036), medical students (p=.0004) and physiotherapy students (p=.0483).

Table 4.6 Descriptive characteristics and tests statistics for differences in respondents' Nutrition Indexes

Nutrition Index[a]	All	students			professionals			
		all	medical	physiotherapy	all	physicians	nurses	physiotherapists
NI12 (Pnt) M ± SD	28.1±3.3	27.9±3.1	28.2±2.9	27.5±3.2	28.5±3.4	29.1±3.2	27.8±3.5	28.5±3.5
NI12								
Low n (%)	262 (33.7)	161 (37.6)	72 (32.3)	89 (43.4)	101 (28.9)	31 (27.9)	42 (36.8)	28 (22.6)
Medium n (%)	250 (32.2)	144 (33.6)	79 (35.4)	65 (31.7)	106 (30.4)	24 (21.6)	35 (30.7)	47 (37.9)
High n (%)	265 (34.1)	123 (28.7)	72 (32.3)	51 (24.9)	142 (40.7)	56 (50.5)	37 (32.5)	49 (39.5)
NI3 (Pnt) M ± SD	6.8 ± 1.6	6.5 ± 1.6	6.8 ± 1.6	6.2 ± 1.6	7.1 ± 1.5	7.1 ± 1.6	6.7 ± 1.6	7.3 ± 1.4
NI3								
Low n (%)	343 (44.1)	218 (50.9)	96 (43.0)	122 (59.5)	125 (35.8)	41 (36.9)	52 (45.6)	32 (25.8)
Medium n (%)	145 (18.7)	79 (18.5)	41 (18.4)	38 (18.5)	66 (18.9)	14 (12.6)	22 (19.3)	30 (24.2)
High n (%)	289 (37.2)	131 (30.6)	86 (38.6)	45 (22.0)	158 (45.3)	56 (50.5)	40 (35.1)	62 (50.0)

	all groups			students/professionals		
	F	p value	η^2	t	p value	Hedges' g
NI12[b]	5.03	.0005	.03	-2.54	.0113	-.185
NI3[b]	11.54	<.0001	.06	-4.89	<.0001	-.349

NI12 – Nutrition Index for 12 dietary behaviour; NI3 – Nutrition Index for 3 dietary behaviour (whole grains, vegetables, fruits);
a – according to nutrition questionnaire results presented in points and divided in 3 categories (STEN);
b – test t or one way ANOVA were used for differences between studied groups; effect size: Hedges' g, eta-squared (η^2)

4.2.3 Smoking

Smoking is one of the most harmful health behaviours. Similar to most European countries, a number of legal measures putting a ban on smoking in public places and advertising of tobacco products in the mass media have been implemented in Poland over the last decade. Still, it is difficult to find any significant improvement in the indices in the past few years. However, we can observe a clear decrease in the percentage of smokers compared to the 1990s.

Table 4.7 Descriptive characteristics and test statistics for differences in respondents' smoking behaviour

		students			professionals		
Smoking	**All**	**all**	**medical**	**physio-therapy**	**all**	**physi-cians**	**nurses**	**physio-therapists**
Current n (%)	145 (18.7)	60 (14.1)	34 (15.4)	26 (12.7)	85 (24.4)	20 (18.0)	36 (31.9)	29 (23.4)
Ex n (%)	81 (10.5)	34 (8.0)	20 (9.1)	14 (6.8)	47 (13.5)	16 (14.4)	12 (10.6)	19 (15.3)
Never n (%)	548 (70.8)	332 (77.9)	167 (75.6)	165 (80.5)	216 (62.1)	75 (67.6)	65 (57.5)	76 (61.3)

	all groups			students/professionals		
	Chi-square	p value	V	Chi-square	p value	V
Smoking[a]	32.64	.00007	.15	23.33	.00001	.17

a - Chi-squared test were used for differences between studied groups; effect size: Cramér's V

Medical service workers play a significant role in prevention programmemes and that's why it is particularly important how they manage this bad habit themselves. Table 7 shows the attitude to smoking of students and medical professionals included in the study. The studied groups vary in terms of intensity of the occurrence of this habit (p<.0001, Cramér's V=.15). The percentage of smokers is highest among nurses and physiotherapists. Every third nurse included in the study smokes on a regular basis – this percentage is higher than the average for women in Poland (Stan zagrożenia epidemią palenia tytoniu w Polsce, 2009). Given their important role in the process of patient education, it is particularly alarming information. We can also notice a higher percentage of regular smokers among current professionals compared to medical students (p<.0001, Cramér's V=.17). The students, preparing for their professional roles, show much more common sense when it comes to their attitude to smoking. Therefore, we might be slightly optimistic about their future without cigarettes. Gender differentiates individual groups of respondents in terms of their attitude to smoking. Such differences can be observed among physicians where men are more frequent smokers (p=.0268, Cramér's V=.26) and among medical students where men also smoke more often than women (p=.0075, Cramér's V=.21).

4.2.4 Alcohol Consumption

Polish traditions and experience related to the patterns of alcohol consumption have not been beneficial to health. Similar to other post-communist, so-called eastern block countries, alcohol in Poland was consumed mainly in the form of high-proof alcoholic beverages and in large quantities. Social and political changes have contributed to a slow change in the patterns and "trends" related to the alcohol use. The consumption of low-proof alcoholic beverages (mainly beer but also wine) has increased while the use of high-proof alcohol (e.g. vodka) has dropped – this issue is discussed in more detail in Chapter 3. Based on the WHO recommendations, the patterns of alcohol consumption by the respondents were classified into four groups: binge, heavy, moderate, abstinent. The percentage values for individual alcohol consumption patterns among the respondents can be found in Table 4.8.

Table 4.8 Descriptive characteristics and tests statistics for differences in respondents' alcohol consumption

Alcohol		students			professionals			
	All	all	medical	physio-therapy	all	physi-cians	nurses	physio-therapists
Binge n (%)	28 (3.6)	16 (3.7)	11 (4.9)	5 (2.4)	12 (3.4)	0 (0)	0 (0)	12 (9.7)
High n (%)	185 (23.8)	126 (29.5)	73 (32.7)	53 (25.9)	59 (16.9)	23 (20.7)	10 (8.8)	26 (21.0)
Medium n (%)	495 (63.7)	242 (56.5)	109 (48.9)	133 (64.9)	253 (72.5)	85 (76.6)	86 (75.4)	82 (66.1)
Abstinent n(%)	69 (8.9)	44 (10.3)	30 (13.5)	14 (6.8)	25 (7.2)	3 (2.7)	18 (15.8)	4 (3.2)

	all groups			students/professionals		
	Chi-square	p value	V	Chi-square	p value	V
Alcohol[a]	76.97	<.0001	.18	22.51	<.0001	.17

a - Chi-squared test were used for differences between studied groups; effect size: Cramer's V

The groups of respondents vary in the frequency of occurrence of individual alcohol consumption categories (p<.0001, Cramér's V=.18). As far as this behaviour is concerned, the worst scores were obtained by the both groups of students and physiotherapists in the case of whom both heavy and binge alcohol consumption are particularly frequent patterns. On the other hand, nurses are a professional group which is least likely to implement adverse patterns of alcohol consumption. As for differences between students and professionals, we can also observe an opposite trend compared to smoking. This time, it is the students who more often demonstrate a level of alcohol use that is detrimental to health (p<.0001, Cramér's V=.17). Gender differentiates the patterns of alcohol consumption in the whole studied group (p<.0001, Cramér's V=.18) where an excessive consumption is observed more frequently among men and similar differences of the average effect size can be observed among medical students (p<.0001, Cramér's V=.30).

4.2.5 Search for the Weakest Link

The analysis of health behaviours in the studied groups of both current and future medical service workers showed considerable differences between them. Each of the evaluated groups has different strengths and weaknesses in their lifestyles. Figures 4.4 and 4.5 present the percentages of both beneficial and adverse patterns of health behaviours implemented by the respondents. As a result, it is possible to identify specific areas requiring educational and promotional intervention with regard to the respondents.

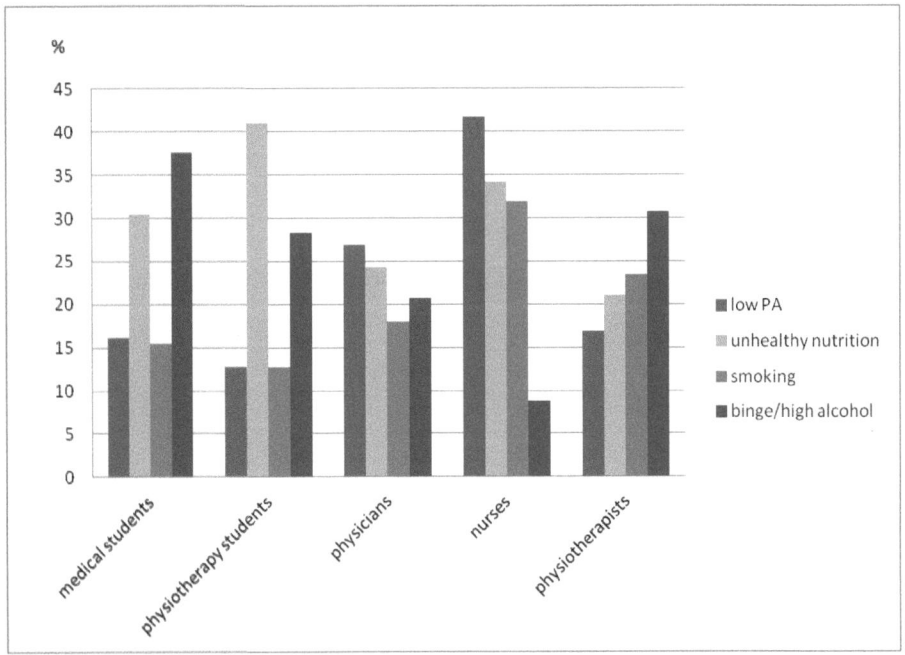

Figure 4.4 The weakest links in the chain of the studied health behaviours of the respondents (in percentages of respondents)

Figure 4.4 clearly shows that nurses are a professional group particularly vulnerable to health effects of their adverse behaviours. For three out of the four studied behaviours at least one in three demonstrates adverse behaviours. The weakest link in the studied behaviours of nurses is their low physical activity. The biggest problem amongst physicians participating in the study is also a sedentary lifestyle. One in four also demonstrate low levels of physical activity. On the other hand, the biggest challenge for physiotherapists is their heavy and excessive consumption of alcohol. Almost one in three exhibits this problem. Improper nutrition is the main problem among physiotherapy students. Over 40% of the respondents demonstrate adverse eating habits. A dominant problem among medical students is that of an excessive consumption of alcohol. Almost 40% of them declared particularly adverse patterns within that scope.

Each of the four social and professional groups demonstrate different weakest links in the chain of health behaviours, and consequently, there are slightly different priourities from the perspective of health promotion.

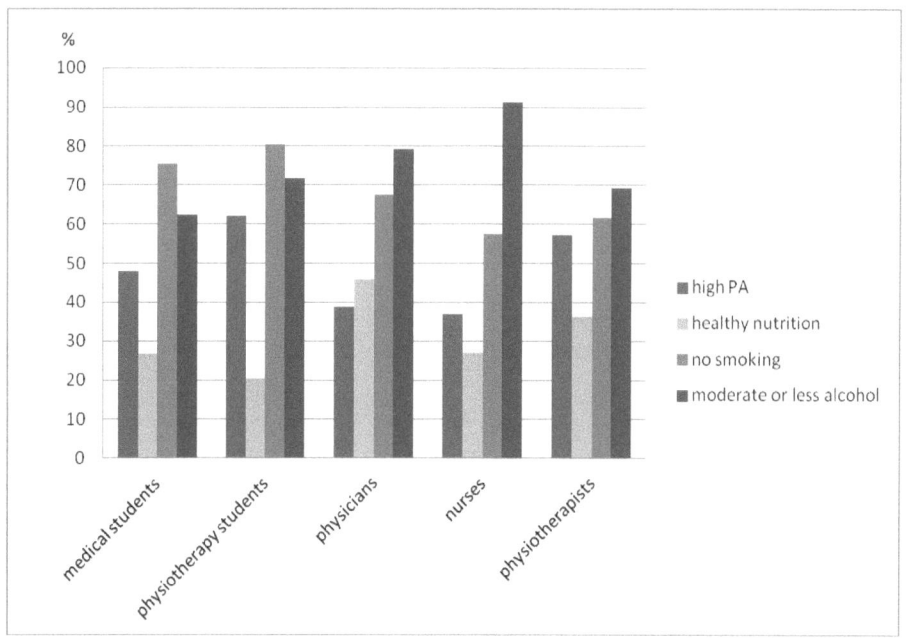

Figure 4.5 The strongest links in the chain of the studied health behaviours of the respondents (in percentages of respondents)

Figure 4.5 presents the percentages of the respondents implementing particularly health-beneficial patterns of behaviour. Here, we can also observe differences between the groups. The vast majority of nurses participating in the study (over 90%) do not abuse alcohol. Most physicians and a considerable part of physiotherapists also implement health recommendations concerning this behaviour. On the other hand, non-smoking is a strength of the studied group of students (almost 80%).

4.2.6 Co-Occurrence of Analysed Health Behaviours

To be able to develop multiple behaviour interventions, one needs to develop a better understanding of the complex relationships among multiple risk behaviours (Stretcher, 2002). In the present study, we attempted to understand the interrelationships between four health risk behaviours – physical activity, nutrition, tobacco use, and alcohol use – among health students and professionals.

At the next stage, patterns of accumulation of the studied health behaviours were sought. Percentages of persons who accumulate adverse or beneficial health behaviours were determined (see Fig. 4.6 and 4.7). Furthermore, percentages of persons following a respective number of the studied health behaviours at the level beneficial to health (from 0 to 4 possible) or destructive to health were determined.

Differences between the studied groups as for the frequency of accumulation of both adverse (p=.0018, Cramér's V=.11) and beneficial (p<.0001, Cramér's V=.13) behaviours were observed. A similar difference can be observed between students and professionals as for the accumulation of adverse (p=.0048, Cramér's V=.14) and beneficial (p<.0001, Cramér's V=.18) behaviours. Generally, we can see a more frequent occurrence of accumulation of adverse behaviours among medical professionals. Nurses compare particularly unfavorably in this regard. Interestingly, a slightly more frequent occurrence of accumulation of all the behaviours beneficial to health can be observed among medical professionals (physiotherapists and physicians in particular). While comparing medical students to physiotherapy students, we can see both less frequent accumulation of beneficial behaviours and more frequent accumulation of adverse behaviours in the first group. Gender does not differentiate the respondents in terms of accumulation of both beneficial and adverse behaviours.

In order to make a more thorough analysis of the co-occurrence of individual health behaviours and their interactions cluster analyses were performed. Four distinct clusters were identified based on four lifestyle risk factors: physical activity, nutrition, smoking and alcohol consumption. The following indicators of behaviours were chosen: two levels of physical activity: low or moderate and high; sum of points for NI12 for nutrition; three levels for smoking: current smoking, ex-smoking, never smoking; two levels for alcohol consumption: moderate and heavy or binge drinking. Four clusters were found to be the optimum number of clusters. Table 4.9 presents the size and features of the distinguished clusters.

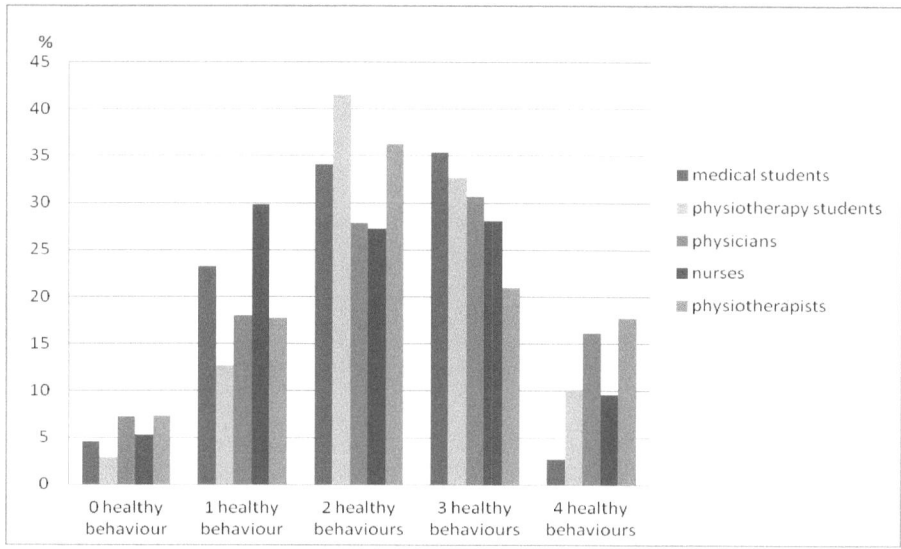

Figure 4.6 Accumulation of healthy behaviours (percentages of respondents)

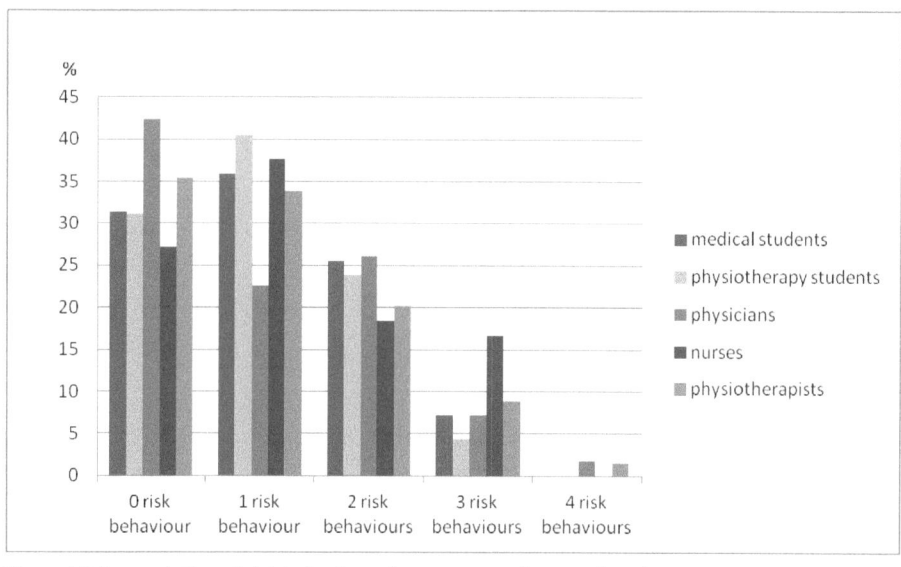

Figure 4.7 Accumulation of risk behaviours (percentages of respondents)

Table 4.9 Descriptive characteristics for each cluster

	Clusters					p value, effect size
	1 unhealthy	2 healthy	3 unhealthy	4 moderate healthy	All	
N (%)	212 (28)	204 (27)	132 (17.5)	208 (27.5)		
NI12 M ± SD	27.8 ± 3.0	29.1 ± 3.1[a]	27.4 ± 3.9[b]	28.1 ± 3.2[b]	28.2 ± 3.3	$p < .0001$, $\eta^2 = .04$
PA (%)		a	b	a, b, c		
low/ moderate	24.0	0	19.9	56.1	49.1	$p < .0001$, $V = .60$
high	31.9	53	15.1	0	50.9	
Smoking (%)		a	a, b	a, c		
never	24.4	37.4	0	38.2	72	$p < .0001$, $V = .59$
ex	26.6	0	73.4	0	10.5	
current	43.9	0	56.1	0	17.5	
Alcohol (%)		a	a	a		
moderate	0	37.5	24.3	38.2	28.0	$p < .0001$, $V = 1.00$
heavy/ binge	100	0	0	0	72	

a – difference from cluster 1 using Bonfernoniego test, chi-squared test or Fisher's exact test for categorical values

b – difference from cluster 2 using Bonfernoniego, test, chi-squared test or Fisher's exact test for categorical values

c – difference from cluster 3 using Bonfernoniego test, chi-squared test or Fisher's exact test for categorical values

Three clusters include 28% of individuals from the sample. The smallest cluster includes 17.5% of persons. Cluster 1 is characterized by heavy or binge drinking status and quite poor diet, i.e. it contains people following adverse lifestyle behaviours. Clusters 2 and 4 are characterized by relatively beneficial nutrition behaviours, moderate consumption of alcohol and non-smoking but they differ in terms of physical activity, where for cluster 4 it can be considered as moderate whereas for cluster 2 as beneficial. Cluster 3 contains current smokers, moderate drinkers with quite poor diet and varying physical activity, i.e. it groups persons adopting adverse lifestyle. The analysed behaviours significantly differentiated individual clusters: physical activity (chi-squared $(3,756)=419.3$, $p < .0001$, Cramér's $V=.60$), smoking (chi-squared $(6,756)=523.5$, $p < .0001$, Cramér's $V=.59$), alcohol (chi-squared $(3,756)=756.0$, $p < .0001$, Cramér's $V=1.00$), nutrition (F $(3,756)=8.8$, $p < .0001$, eta squared$=.04$). We can observe also differences between individual clusters in terms of the percentage of persons representing given behaviours or averages characterizing them (see Tab. 4.9).

Individual clusters differ from each other as for the representation of the analysed career stage groups: professionals and students (chi-squared (3,756)=38.0, p<.0001, Cramér's V=.22). The difference is particularly visible in cluster 1 and cluster 3. Cluster 1, containing persons abusing alcohol with adverse nutrition behaviours, consists mostly of students whereas cluster 3, containing persons with poor diet, not abusing alcohol and currently smoking or ex-smoking, consists mostly of professionals (see Fig. 4.8).

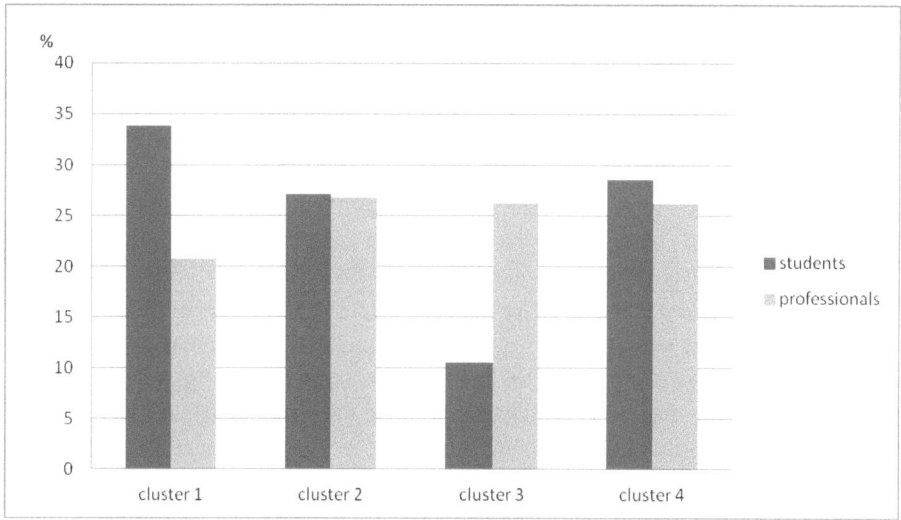

Figure 4.8 Representation of students and professionals in clusters (percentages)

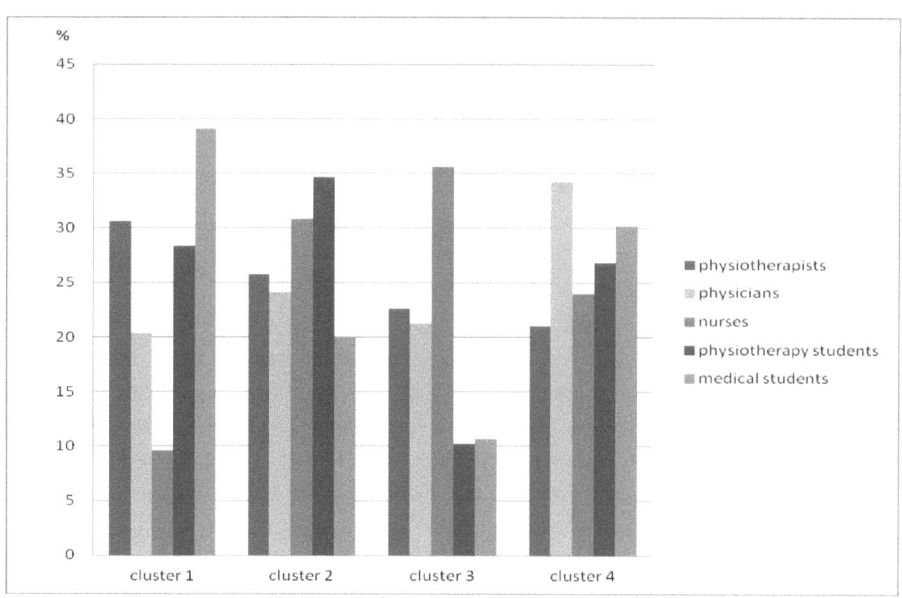

Figure 4.9 Representation of each studied groups in clusters (percentages)

Similarly, the five surveyed social and professional groups vary in the frequency of representation of individual clusters (chi-squared (12,156)=72.63, p<.0001, Cramér's V=.18). The cluster most frequently represented among physiotherapists is cluster 1, among physicians cluster 4, among nurses cluster 3, among physiotherapy students cluster 2 and among medical students cluster 1 (see Fig. 4.9). Gender does not differentiate the respondents in respect of the frequency of belonging to individual clusters.

Next, differences were sought between persons assigned to the distinguished clusters in terms of the following subject variables: health locus of control, place of health as a personal value, self-rated health and BMI. Both a chi-squared test and an analysis of variance were used for that purpose. The respondents from the individual clusters differed in self-rated health (chi-squared (12,747)=43.35, p<.0001, Cramér's V=.14). The respondents rating their health as very bad, bad or moderate are more rarely represented in cluster 2 which is more often represented by persons rating their health as very good. On the other hand, cluster 3 is more rarely represented by persons rating their health as good and very good and relatively often by persons rating their health as moderate or worse. The valuation of health as a prerequisite for happiness does not differentiate the respondents in terms of belonging to particular clusters (chi-squared (15,756)=17.44, p=.2912, Cramér's V=.09). However, the respondents differ in the perception of health as an important, personal value (chi-squared (15,756)=29.57, p=.0143, Cramér's V=.11). The persons who do not value health more often represent cluster 1 or cluster 3, whereas persons who appreciate the value of health more often represent cluster 2 and cluster 4. As for health locus of control, we can see the following differences between the distinguished clusters. Internal Health Locus Of Control differentiates the respondents (chi-squared (3,755)=8.74, p=.0333, Cramér's V=.11). The respondents with high Internal Health Locus of Control, i.e. believing that the state of their health depends on them most frequently represent cluster 2. The respondents with low belief in that regard more frequently represent clusters 1 and 4. Similarly, others health locus of control differentiates the respondents in the distinguished clusters (chi-squared (3,755)=12.91, p=.0047, Cramér's V=.13). The persons placing control over their own health in the hands of health specialist more frequently represent clusters 1 and 4 whereas the persons who do not entrust the control over their health to specialist can be more frequently found in cluster 2. Also the third type, Chance Health Locus of Control differentiates the respondents (chi-squared (3,755)=9.60, p=.0221, Cramér's V=.11). The respondents with low Chance Health Locus of Control more often represent cluster 1 whereas those with high Chance Health Locus of Control, i.e. entrusting control over their health to chance, fate or God more frequently represent cluster 4.

The analysis focused also on differences in the BMI category between the respondents representing individual clusters (chi-squared (39,744)=41.21, p<.0001, Cramér's V=.14). The overweight respondents most frequently represent cluster 3, persons with normal body weight represent cluster 2 whereas underweight persons represent clusters 1 and 4.

The study focused also on the analysis of how the individual behaviours (nutrition, smoking, alcohol consumption), affiliation to one of the studied social and professional groups and their interaction differentiate a level of physical activity among the respondents. For that purpose, a two-way analysis of variance was employed and the percentage of explained variation for the variable "level of physical activity" by the aforementioned factors was determined. The results are presented in graphs.

A relationship between nutrition behaviour (for both NI12 and NI3), professional career stage or affiliation to one of the studied groups and a level of physical activity of the respondents was subject of analysis. The main effects of NI12 and career stage and the effect of interaction (NI12 x career stage) are significant (p<.0001). Students declare a higher level of physical activity than professionals (p<.0001). The respondents demonstrating beneficial nutrition behaviour have physical activity score higher than those with adverse nutrition behaviour (p=.0011). The level of nutrition does not differentiate physical activity among students but it does among professionals. The professionals demonstrating adverse nutrition behaviours have physical activity score significantly lower than those with moderate (p<.0001) and beneficial (p<.0001) nutrition behaviours. The career stage differentiates a level of physical activity only among those with adverse nutrition behaviours – physical activity of students is higher than that of professionals (p<.0001). In the whole group professionals with adverse nutrition behaviours compare unfavorably, demonstrating a level of physical activity significantly lower than that of all the other respondents (p<.0001). The model explains 8% of the variance in the dependent variable (F(5,762)=13.24, p<.0001, R^2=.08) – see Figure 4.10.

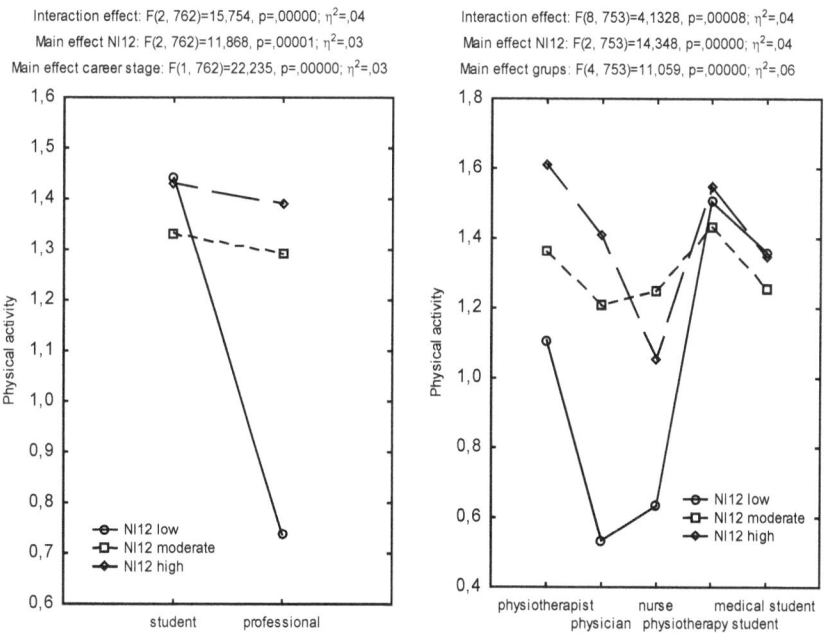

Figure 4.10 NI12, physical activity and career stage or studied groups interaction (two-way ANOVA results)

The main effects of NI12 and group and the effect of interaction (NI12 x group) are significant (p<.0001). The respondents demonstrating beneficial nutrition behaviours have physical activity score significantly higher than those with adverse nutrition behaviours (p=.0009). A level of physical activity of both physiotherapists and physiotherapy students is significantly higher than that of physicians and nurses (p<.05). The nutrition behaviour differentiates a level of physical activity among physicians and nurses. The physicians demonstrating adverse nutrition behaviours have physical activity score significantly lower than those with beneficial nutrition behaviours (p=.0001). The nurses demonstrating moderate nutrition behaviours have physical activity score significantly higher than those with adverse nutrition behaviours (p=.0382). The biggest differences between the social and professional groups can be observed among persons demonstrating adverse nutrition behaviours. The model explains 10% of the variance in the dependent variable (F(14,753)=6.8, p<.0001, R^2=.10) – see Figure 4.10.

The same procedure was carried out for NI3. The main effects of NI3 and career stage and the effect of interaction (NI3 x career stage) are significant (p<.0001). Students declare a higher level of physical activity than professionals (p<.0001). The respondents demonstrating adverse nutrition behaviours have physical activity score significantly lower than those with moderate (p=.0046) and beneficial (p=.0001) nutrition behaviours. The level of nutrition does not differentiate physical activity among students but it does among professionals. The professionals demonstrating adverse nutrition behaviours have physical activity score significantly lower than those with moderate (p<.0001) and beneficial (p<.0001) nutrition behaviours. The career stage most often differentiates a level of physical activity among those with adverse nutrition behaviours – physical activity of students is higher than that of professionals (p<.0001). In the whole group professionals with adverse nutrition behaviours compare unfavorably, demonstrating a level of physical activity significantly lower than that of the other respondents (p<.0001). The model explains 9% of the variance in the dependent variable (F(5,762)=15.31, p<.0001, R^2=.09) – see Figure 4.11.

The main effects of NI3 and group and the effect of interaction (NI3 x group) are significant (p=.0020). The respondents demonstrating adverse nutrition behaviours have physical activity score significantly lower than those with moderate (p=.0040) and beneficial (p<.0001) nutrition behaviours. A level of physical activity of both physiotherapists and physiotherapy students is significantly higher than that of physicians and nurses (p<.05). The nutrition behaviour differentiates a level of physical activity among physiotherapists, physicians and nurses. The physiotherapists demonstrating adverse nutrition behaviours have physical activity score significantly lower than those with beneficial nutrition behaviours (p=.0093). The physicians demonstrating adverse nutrition behaviours have physical activity scores significantly lower than those with beneficial nutrition behaviours (p=.0143). The nurses demonstrating adverse nutrition behaviours have also physical activity scores significantly lower than those with beneficial nutrition behaviours (p=.0032). The biggest differences between the social and professional groups can be observed among persons demonstrating adverse nutrition behaviours. The model explains 11% of the variance in the dependent variable (F(14,753)=7.50, p<.0001, R^2=.11) – see Figure 4.11.

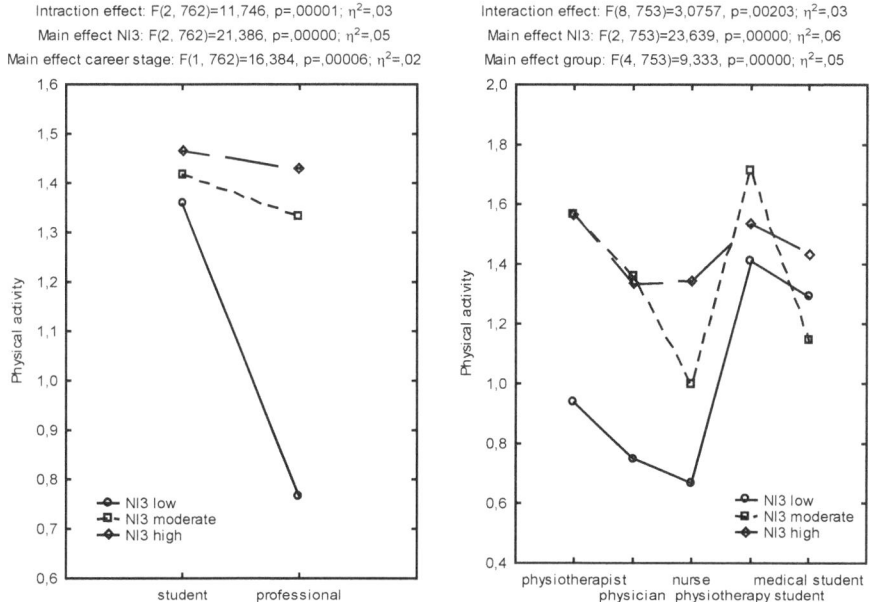

Figure 4.11 NI3, physical activity and career stage or studied groups interaction (two-way ANOVA results)

Furthermore, the study focused on the analysis of a relationship between smoking, professional career stage or affiliation to one of the studied groups and a level of physical activity of the respondents. The main effect of career stage and the effect of interaction (smoking x career stage) are significant (p<.0001, p=.0055, respectively). The effect of smoking proved to be insignificant. Students declare a higher level of physical activity (p<.0001). Smoking does not differentiate a level of physical activity among students whereas smoking professionals have significantly lower activity score than non-smoking ones (p=.0012). The career stage differentiates a level of physical activity mainly among smokers. Smoking students declare a higher level of physical activity than professionals (p=.0003). Generally, as for physical activity, smoking professionals compare particularly unfavorably to almost all the other groups (p<.002), except for ex-smoking professionals. The model explains 4% of the variance in the dependent variable (F(5,759)=6.62, p<.0001, R^2=.04) – see Figure 4.12.

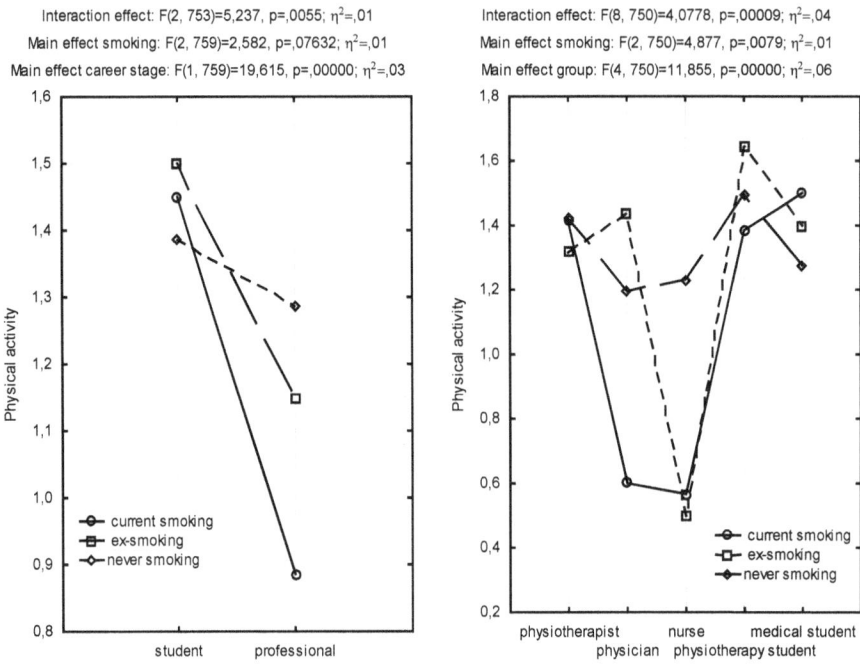

Interaction effect: F(2, 753)=5,237, p=,0055; η²=,01
Main effect smoking: F(2, 759)=2,582, p=,07632; η²=,01
Main effect career stage: F(1, 759)=19,615, p=,00000; η²=,03

Interaction effect: F(8, 750)=4,0778, p=,00009; η²=,04
Main effect smoking: F(2, 750)=4,877, p=,0079; η²=,01
Main effect group: F(4, 750)=11,855, p=,00000; η²=,06

Figure 4.12 Smoking, physical activity and career stage or studied groups interaction (two-way ANOVA results)

The main effects of smoking and group and the effect of interaction (smoking x group) are significant (p<.0001, p=.0079, p=.0001, respectively). The level of physical activity of both physiotherapists and physiotherapy students is significantly higher than that of physicians and nurses (p<.04). Physical activity of smokers is significantly lower than that of non-smokers (p=.0068). Smoking differentiates a level of physical activity only among nurses where smokers have significantly lower physical activity score than non-smokers (p=.0059). On the other hand, social and professional groups differentiate physical activity most often among smokers. Smoking physicians and nurses have physical activity scores significantly lower than smoking physiotherapists, medicine and physiotherapy students (p<.04). Generally, smoking nurses have the worst score with physical activity significantly lower (p<.01) compared to all the other non-smoking respondent groups and ex-smokers (except for nurses who gave up smoking). On the other hand, smoking physicians have physical activity score significantly lower than smoking and ex-smoking physiotherapy students as well as non-smoking physiotherapists and medical students (p<.01). The model explains 8% of the variance in the dependent variable (F(14,750)=5.82, p<.0001, R²=.08) – see Figure 4.12.

The main effects of alcohol and career stage and the effect of interaction (alcohol x career stage) are insignificant. The main effects of alcohol and group are significant (p=.0242, p=.0002, respectively). The effect of interaction (alcohol x group) proved to be insignificant. Moderate drinkers have higher physical activity score than those with heavy alcohol consumption (p=.0063). The model explains 5% of the variance in the dependent variable (F(14,753)=4.10, p<.0001, R^2=.05) – see Figure 4.13.

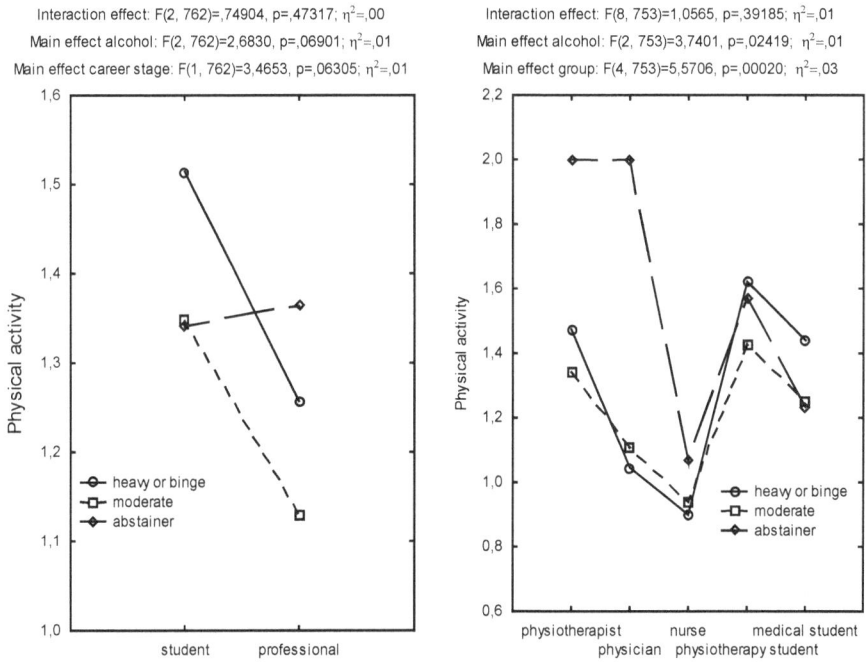

Figure 4.13 Alcohol consumption, physical activity and career stage or studied groups interaction (two-way ANOVA results)

Next, the study focused on the analysis of a relationship between alcohol consumption, professional career stage or affiliation to one of the studied groups and nutrition behaviour of the respondents. The main effects of alcohol and career stage and the interaction (alcohol x career stage) are insignificant. These factors do not differentiate nutrition behaviour (NI12) of the respondents. On the other hand, the main effects of alcohol and group and the interaction (alcohol x group) are significant (p<.03). Physiotherapy students demonstrate a significantly worse nutrition behaviour than physiotherapists (p=.0373) or physicians (p=.0003) whereas nurses' nutrition behaviour is worse than that of physicians (p=.0343). The consumption of alcohol differentiates nutrition behaviour only among nurses where, interestingly, drinking or abstinent respondents rarely demonstrate a significantly worse nutrition behaviour than moderately drinking ones (p=.0472). However, social and professional groups do not differentiate nutrition behaviour among those with heavy or binge alcohol consumption. There is minimal difference between the other alcohol consumption groups. The biggest difference can be found between abstinent nurses demonstrating a significantly worse nutrition behaviour than moderately drinking physiotherapists (p=.0108), physicians (p=.0022) and nurses (p=.0472) as well as abstinent students (p=.0239). The model explains 4% of the variance in the dependent variable ($F(14,762)=3.54$, $p<.0001$, $R^2=.04$) – see Figure 4.14.

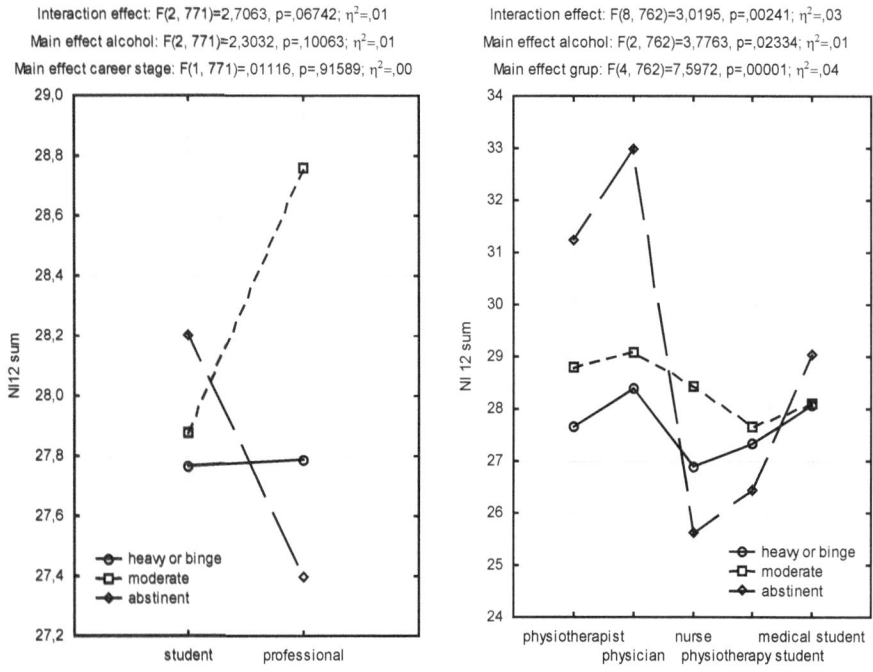

Figure 4.14 Alcohol consumption, nutrition status (NI12) and career stage or studied groups interaction (two-way ANOVA results).

The main effect of career stage and the interaction (alcohol x career stage) are significant ($p<.04$). These factors differentiate nutrition behaviour (NI3) of the respondents. The main effect of alcohol proved to be insignificant. Professionals demonstrate a significantly better nutrition behaviour than students ($p<.0001$). The consumption of alcohol does not differentiate nutrition behaviours in the group of students and professionals. A distinguishing group here includes moderately drinking professionals with nutrition behaviour significantly better than that of students with heavy, binge or moderate alcohol consumption ($p<.003$).

The model explains 3% of the variance in the NI3 dependent variable (F(5,771)=36.31, p<.0001, R^2=.03) – see Figure 4.15.

The main effect of group and the effect of interaction (alcohol x group) are significant (p<.02). These factors differentiate nutrition behaviour (NI3) of the respondents. The main effect of alcohol proved to be insignificant. Physiotherapist demonstrate significantly better nutrition behaviour than nurses (p=.0462), physiotherapy students (p<.0001) and medical students (p=.0214). Physiotherapy students demonstrate significantly worse nutrition behaviour than physicians (p<.0001) and medical students (p=.0017) and better than nurses (p=.0271). The level of alcohol consumption does not differentiate nutrition behaviours in the studied groups of respondents. A distinguishing group here includes moderately drinking physiotherapists and physicians with nutrition behaviour significantly better than that of physiotherapy students with rare or moderate (p<.005) and heavy or binge (p<.0105) alcohol consumption. The model explains 7% of the variance in the NI3 dependent variable (F(14,762)=4.87, p<.0001, R^2=.07) – see Figure 4.15.

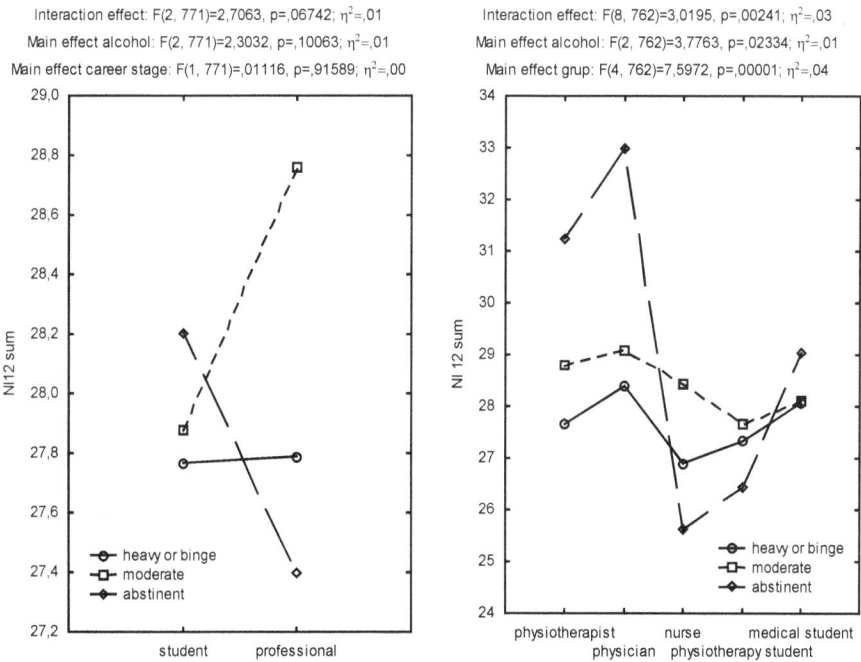

Figure 4.15 Alcohol consumption, nutrition status (NI3) and career stage or studied groups interaction (two-way ANOVA results)

Below, a relationship between smoking, professional career stage or affiliation to one of the studied groups and nutrition behaviour of the respondents (NI12 and NI3) was analysed.

The main effect of career stage is insignificant. The main effect of smoking and the effect of interaction (smoking x career stage) are significant (p<.01). These factors differentiate nutrition behaviour (NI12) of the respondents. Current smokers demonstrate a significantly worse nutrition behaviour than ex-smokers (p=.0012) and non-smokers (p<.0001). Professionals demonstrate a significantly better nutrition behaviour than students (p<.0001). Smoking differentiates nutrition behaviour only among professionals. Smoking professionals demonstrate a significantly worse nutrition behaviour than their colleagues who are ex-smokers (p=.0012) and non-smokers (p<.0001). A distinguishing group here includes non-smoking professionals with nutrition behaviour significantly better than that of smoking students (p<.003) as well as both non-smoking (p<.0001) and smoking (p<.0001) professionals. Ex-smoking professionals demonstrate also a better nutrition behaviour than smoking ones (p<.0012). The model explains 6% of the variance in the NI12 dependent variable (F(5,768)=11.36, p<.0001, R^2=.06) – see Figure 4.16.

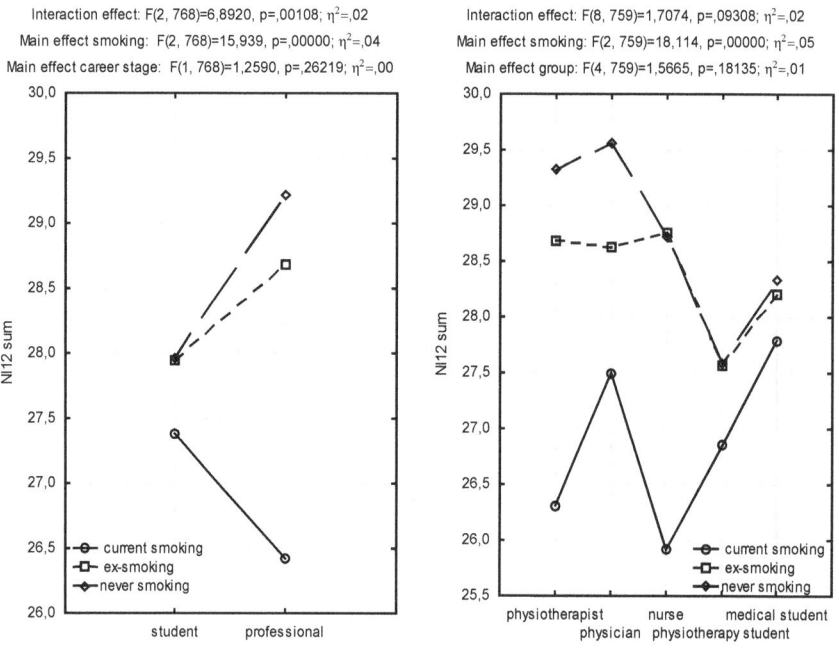

Figure 4.16 Smoking, nutrition status (NI12) and career stage or studied groups interaction (two-way ANOVA results)

The main effect of group and the effect of interaction (smoking x group) are insignificant. These factors do not differentiate nutrition behaviour (NI12) of the respondents. The main effect of smoking proved to be significant (p<.0001). Smokers demonstrate a significantly worse nutrition behaviour than ex-smokers (p=.0011) and non-smokers (p<.0001). The model explains 7% of the variance in the NI12 dependent variable (F(14,759)=4.94, p<.0001, R^2=.07) – see Figure 4.16.

The main effects of smoking and career stage and the effect of interaction (smoking x career stage) are significant (p<.02). These factors differentiate nutrition behaviour (NI3) of the respondents. Current smokers demonstrate a significantly worse nutrition behaviour than ex-smokers (p=.0001) and non-smokers (p<.0198) whereas, interestingly, nutrition behaviour of non-smokers is worse than that of ex-smokers (p=.0071). Professionals demonstrate a significantly better nutrition behaviour than students (p<.0001). Smoking differentiates nutrition behaviour only among professionals. Smoking professionals demonstrate a significantly worse nutrition behaviour than their colleagues who are ex-smokers (p=.0038) and non-smokers (p<.0003). It is only in the group of non-smokers that students demonstrate worse nutrition behaviour than professionals (p<.0001). A distinguishing group here includes non-smoking professionals with nutrition behaviour significantly better than that of both smoking (p<.003) and non-smoking (p<.0001) students as well as smoking professionals (p<.00001). Ex-smoking professionals demonstrate also a better nutrition behaviour than smoking ones (p<.0012). The model explains 6% of the variance in the NI3 dependent variable (F(5,768)=10.77, p<.0001, R^2=.06) – see Figure 4.17.

The main effects of smoking (p<.0001) and group are significant (p=.0045). These factors differentiate nutrition behaviour (NI3) of the respondents. The effect of interaction (smoking x group) is insignificant. Physiotherapy students demonstrate significantly worse nutrition behaviour in all the studied groups (p<.02) whereas nutrition behaviour of medical students is worse than that of physiotherapists (p=.0231). Smokers demonstrate a significantly worse nutrition behaviour than ex-smokers (p=.0001) and non-smokers (p<.0182) whereas nutrition behaviour of ex-smokers is better than that of non-smokers (p=.0065). The model explains 8% of the variance in the NI3 dependent variable (F(14,759)=5.76, p<.0001, R^2=.08) – see Figure 4.17.

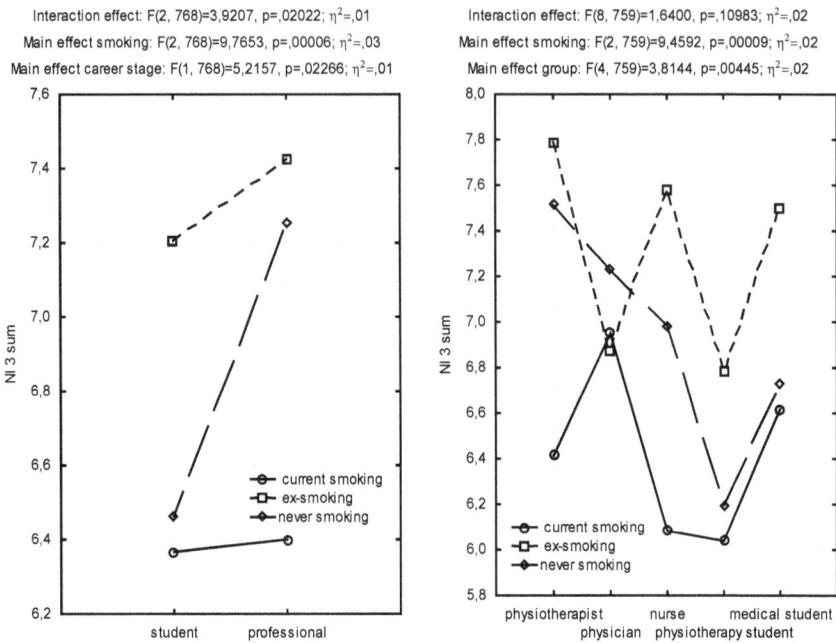

Figure 4.17 Smoking, nutrition status (NI3) and career stage or studied groups interaction (two-way ANOVA results)

4.2.7 Health Behaviour Profiles

In accordance with the procedure described in the methodological part of the study, an original classification of health-related activities was proposed, taking the four studied health behaviours into consideration, including two health-enhancing behaviours and two health-compromising behaviours. Five Health Behaviour Profiles were distinguished: *destructive, passive, ambivalent, average, beneficial.* Descriptive statistics for each profile were designed in Table 4.10.

The frequency of occurrence of individual Health Behaviour Profiles varies between the group of students and the group of professionals (p<.0001, Cramér's V=.18). The *destructive* profile is more common among professionals whereas the *ambivalent* and *average* profiles are more common among students. Differentiation between all the studied groups proved to be significant, albeit of small effect size (p<.0001, Cramér's V=.14). The *destructive* profile is observed in the biggest percentage most frequently among nurses, the *passive* profile among physiotherapists, the *ambivalent* profile among physicians, the *average* profile among medical students and the *beneficial* among physiotherapy students. Gender does not differentiate the respondents in respect of the frequency of the Health Behaviour Profiles represented by them.

Table 4.10 Descriptive statistics for Health Behaviour Profiles

Health Behaviour Profiles	students				professionals			
	All	**all**	**medical**	**physio-therapy**	**all**	**physicians**	**nurses**	**physio-thera-pists**
destructive n(%)	104 (14)	37 (9)	22 (10)	15 (7)	67 (20)	16 (15)	33 (31)	18 (14)
passive n (%)	91 (12)	56 (13)	27 (12)	29 (14)	35 (10)	16 (15)	9 (8)	10 (8)
ambivalent n(%)	94 (12)	54 (13)	32 (15)	22 (11)	40 (12)	12 (11)	6 (6)	22 (18)
average n (%)	154 (20)	101(23)	59 (27)	42 (21)	53 (16)	17 (16)	11 (10)	25 (20)
beneficial n (%)	322 (42)	178(42)	81 (36)	97 (47)	144(42)	47 (43)	48 (45)	49 (40)

	all groups			students/professionals		
	Chi-square	p value	V	Chi-square	p value	V
Health Behaviour Profiles[a]	58.53	<.0001	.14	24.56	<.0001	.18

[a] - *Chi-squared test were used for differences between studied groups; effect size: Cramér's V*

Next, differences between the distinguished Health Behaviour Profiles (HBP) were determined in terms of the following subject variables: health locus of control, place of health as a personal value, self-rated health and BMI. Self-rated health differentiates the respondents representing individual HBPs (chi-squared (16,756)=75.20, p<.0001, Cramér's V=.16). The highest percentage of respondents rating their health as bad or very bad can be observed among the destructive and ambivalent profiles. The persons who most frequently rate their health as very good belong to the beneficial profile (see Fig. 4.18).

The respondents representing individual profiles differ in their valuation of health as a prerequisite for personal happiness (chi-squared (20,765)=49.26, p<.001, Cramér's V=.13). Persons with the destructive and ambivalent profiles most frequently do not regard health as necessary for personal life satisfaction. On the other hand, it is most often highly valued by representatives of the beneficial profile. The situation is quite similar with reference to health as an important, personal value (chi-squared (20,765)=45.96, p=.001, Cramér's V=.12). Most frequently health is not chosen as an important personal value by persons representing the destructive profile while it is perceived as important by persons from the beneficial profile and, interestingly, as very important by persons from the ambivalent profile.

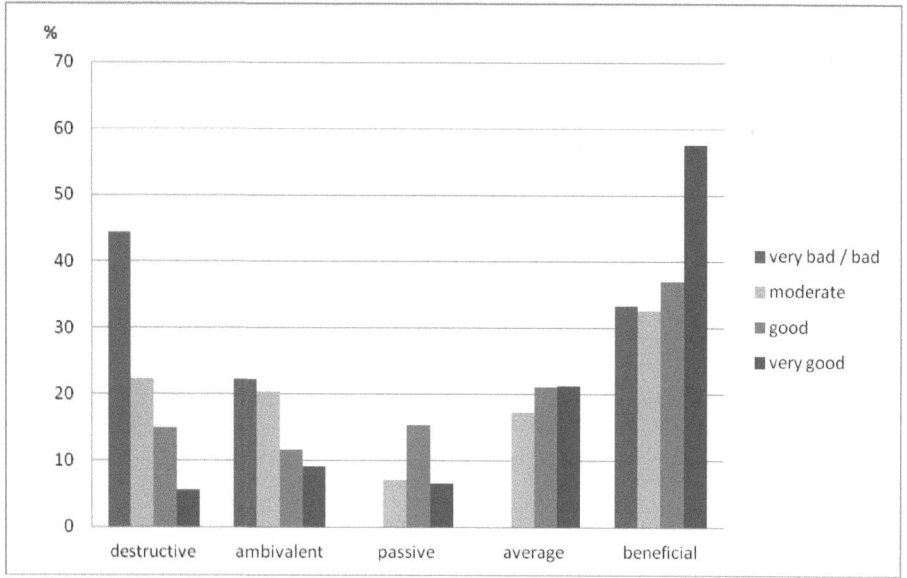

Figure 4.18 Self-rated Health of respondents in each health behaviour profile

Health locus of control also differentiates the respondents. As for Internal Locus Of Health Control (chi-squared (4,764)=24.11, p<.0001, Cramér's V=.18) persons with a high sense of control over their own health most often represent the beneficial and average profiles while persons with low sense of such control represent the destructive, ambivalent and passive profiles (see Fig.4.19). Powerful Others Health Locus of Control did not differentiate the respondents whereas external control related to the role of chance and fate, i.e. Chance Health Locus of Control did differentiate them (chi-squared (4,764)=19.00, p<.001, Cramér's V=.16) but the situation was opposite to that for internal control - persons representing the beneficial, average and ambivalent profiles less frequently give control over their health to the indicated external factors but such control is more often given by representatives of the destructive and passive profiles (see Fig. 4.20).

Also BMI differentiates the respondents representing individual HBPs (chi-squared (12,753)=42.34, p<.0001, Cramér's V=.14). We observe that overweight persons are most often representatives of the destructive profile whereas representatives of the beneficial and average profiles are most frequently those with normal body weight. Underweight can be observed most often among persons representing the average and passive profiles.

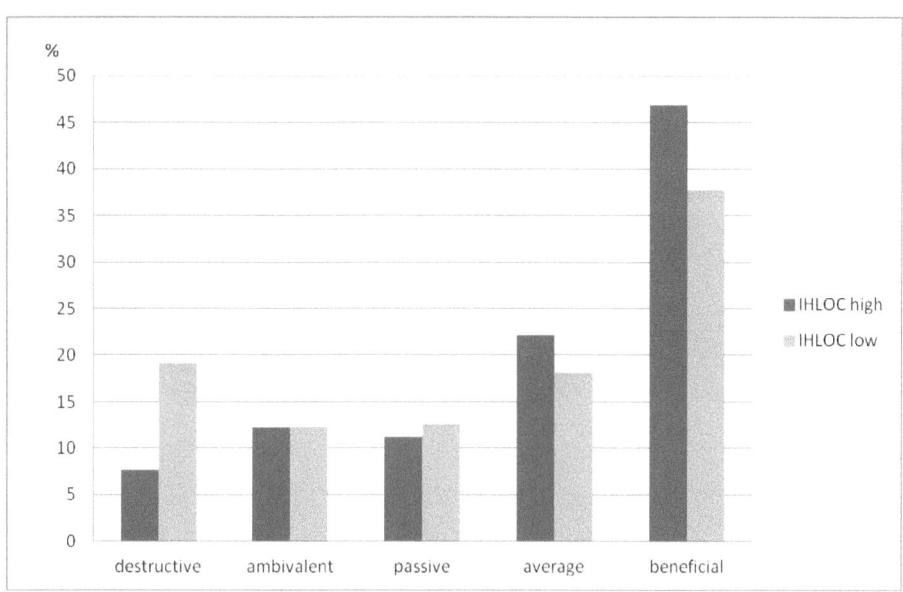

Figure 4.19 Internal Health Locus of Control (IHLOC) differentiation of health behaviours profiles

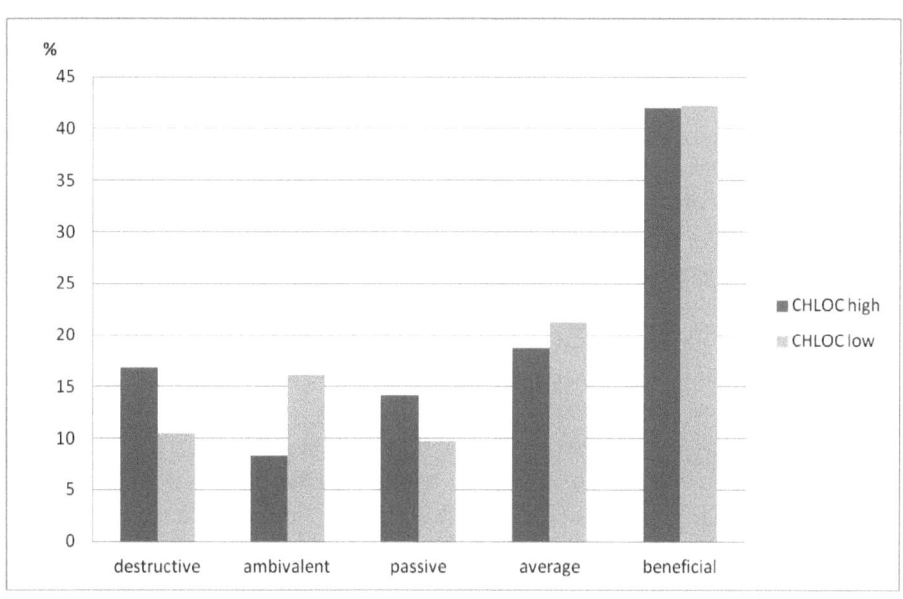

Figure 4.20 Chance Health Locus of Control (CHLOC) differentiation of Health Behaviours Profiles

4.3 Individual Differences Among Medical and Physiotherapy Students and Professionals

During the search for subjective determinants of health behaviours a focus was placed on variables appearing in a number of theories explaining the adoption of a certain lifestyle by an individual. The following were found to be the basic ones: health locus of control, health-specific self-efficacy, health as a personal value, self-rated health. The variations in them within the surveyed social and professional groups are presented in Table 4.11.

Differences in the level of the five distinguished psychosocial determinants were observed between the groups of students and professionals, i.e. in relation to the stage of professional career. For most of the aforementioned variables significantly higher scores were obtained by students: Self-rated Health (p=.026, Glasses' g=.08), physical activity self-efficacy (p=.0004, Hedges' g=.25), nutrition self-efficacy (p=.0012, Hedges' g=.33), Internal Health Locus of Control (p=.014, Hedges' g=.25). Compared to their older professional colleagues, students are more certain of their ability to deal with obstacles to being physically active or to implementing proper diet. Though this conviction does not always go hand in hand with more beneficial behaviours (which is particularly visible in the case of nutrition), you can have an impression that even if they don't adopt health-beneficial behaviours, they still believe that such adoption is mainly up to them and that they can change their habits for the better if only they want to. Maybe they still do not see any need for doing so since, as already mentioned, they have Self-rated Health scores also significantly higher than those of professionals. On the other hand, unsurprisingly, professionals appreciate more the value of health (p<.0001, Glasses' g=.17).

The larger baggage of experience related to the years of work makes them more appreciative of the value of health in life. Furthermore, over all these years they have probably achieved a satisfactory level in respect of other important values and at present they may focus more and more on what often begins to fail with age. Gender differentiates the respondents only in terms of health evaluation as a condition of personal happiness (chi-squared (5,777)=24.56, p<.001, Cramer's V=.18). Women often choose health as an important or very important value in their life more often than men.

While analyzing the position of other values in the hierarchy of values of the respondents, we can see numerous generation differences (see Tab. 4.12).

The hierarchy of values being symbols of personal happiness is similar in the both surveyed groups (Tab. 4.13); however, certain values prove to be important and very important significantly more often to professionals: family (p<.0001, Cramér's V=.17), good health (p=.0009, Cramér's V=.16), doing favorite job (p=004, Cramér's V=.15). On the other hand, other values generally less important to the respondents, prove to be important more often to the group of students: many friends (p<.0001, Cramér's V=.19), being needed by others (p=.0092, Cramér's V=.14), good financial situation (p=.0093, Cramér's V=.14). These results are not surprising and they are an

Table 4.11 Descriptive statistics for psychosocial variables

		All	students		professionals			p value[a] / effect size	p value[b] / effect size
			medical	physiotherapy	physicians	nurses	physiotherapists		
MHCL M ± SD	Internal	27.9 ± 4.4	27.8 ± 4.6	28.7 ± 3.9	28.2 ± 4.0	27.2 ± 4.4	27.1 ± 4.9	.014 / .25	.010 / .02
	Powerful	17.3 ± 5.6	17.4 ± 5.7	17.5 ± 4.9	17.0 ± 5.2	18.6 ± 6.6	15.8 ± 5.5	.321 / Ns	.003 / .02
	Change	16.6 ± 5.6	16.2 ± 5.5	17.3 ± 5.2	15.9 ± 5.0	17.7 ± 5.8	16.0 ± 6.3	.578 / Ns	.018 / .02
PA SE	M ± SD	12.4 ± 4.2	12.7 ± 4.3	13.0 ± 3.9	12.6 ± 4.1	10.4 ± 4.1	12.4 ± 4.1	.000 / .25	.000 / .04
Nutrition SE	M ± SD	13.9 ± 3.6	14.3 ± 3.4	14.3 ± 3.1	14.1 ± 4.4	13.2 ± 3.5	13.0 ± 3.8	.001 / .33	.002 / .02
Smoking SE	M ± SD	31.9 ± 7.2	31.6 ± 7.2	32.7 ± 6.7	33.0 ± 6.4	30.2 ± 8.3	31.6 ± 7.2	.276 / Ns	.018 / .02
Alcohol SE	M ± SD	10.2 ± 2.3	11.4 ± 1.4	10.0 ± 2.2	10.1 ± 2.8	10.3 ± 2.0	7.8 ± 3.4	.449 / Ns	.000 / .10
Health as a value	M ± SD	3.4 ± 1.6	3.2 ± 1.5	3.3 ± 1.6	3.2 ± 1.8	4.0 ± 1.4	3.5 ± 1.6	.000 / .17	.000 / .02
Health as a happiness symbol	M ± SD	3.3 ± 1.6	3.3 ± 1.7	3.3 ± 1.6	3.2 ± 1.6	3.9 ± 1.1	3.2 ± 1.4	.594 / .03	.590 / Ns
SRH	M ± SD	4.1 ± .7	4.2 ± .7	4.1 ± .6	4.2 ± .7	3.8 ± .7	4.2 ± .5	.026 / .08	.026 / .001

a – test t or Mann-Whitney U test were used for differences between students/professionals and Hedges' g or Glass' g effect size
b – one-way ANOVA or Kruskal-Wallis test were used for differences between all groups and eta squared or epsilon squared effect size

Table 4.12 List of Personal Values (LPV) – symbols of personal happiness – mean values of importance and distribution of significance for students (S) and professionals (P)

Symbols of happiness	Mean value of importance TOTAL/S/P	SD TOTAL/S/P	Distribution of significance: S (%) / P (%)					
			5	4	3	2	1	0
1. Many friends	1.49/ 1.67/ 1.27	1.7/ 1.7/ 1.6	4/5	13/8	20/12	15/12	5/10	43/53
2. Being needed by others	1.28/ 1.37/ 1,16	1.6/ 1.6/ 1.4	7/3	8/5	9/12	15/13	12/19	49/48
3. Success at work, school	.93/ 1.03/ .81	1.4/ 1.4/ 1.3	4/2	5/5	8/5	13/12	15/12	56/64
4. Good health	3.34/ 3.27/ 3.43	1.6/ 1.7/ 1.4	31/24	24/35	15/20	12/10	9/5	9/6
5. Life full of adventure, journey	.47/ .54/ .38	1.0/ 1.1/ 0.9	½/2	3/0	3/2	4/4	17/13	72/79
6. Successful family life	3.94/ 3.82/ 4.09	1.4/ 1.4/ 1.4	41/54	32/28	10/5	7/3	6/4	4/6
7. Good financial situation	1.18/ 1.23/ 1.13	1.4/ 1.5/ 1.3	6/2	5/4	11/11	10/15	19/24	49/44
8. Fame, celebrity	.02/ .00/ .04	0.3/ 0.0/ 0.4	0/1	0/0	0/0	0/0	0/0	100/99
9. Doing favourite job	2.03/ 1.95/ 2.14	1.5/ 1.5/ 1.4	6/3	9/12	23/29	21/27	17/10	24/19

S-students; P-professionals; Distribution: 5 – the most important value; 0 – not selected

Table 4.13 List of Personal Values (LPV) – personal values - mean values and distribution of significance for students (S) and professionals (P)

Personal values	Mean value of importance TOTAL/S/P	SD TOTAL/S/P	Distribution of significance S (%) / P (%)					
			5	4	3	2	1	0
1. Love, friendship	3.90/3.98/3.81	1.6 / 1.6 / 1.6	61/51	16/22	4/5	3/7	12/7	5/7
2. Good health	3.38/3.22/3.57	1.6 / 1.6 / 1.6	19/32	39/39	12/6	12/7	7/5	10/10
3. Joy, satisfaction	1.72/1.79/1.62	1.6 / 1.6 / 1.5	4/4	12/10	22/15	16/20	12/14	34/36
4. Sense of humour	.85/.83/.87	1.3 / 1.3 / 1.4	2/3	4/2	8/13	9/8	15/11	62/63
5. Knowledge, wisdom	1.29/1.22/1.38	1.5 / 1.5 / 1.4	4/1	4/6	15/20	15/15	9/15	53/42
6. Attractiveness, appearance	.29/.33/.25	0.8 / 0.9 / 0.7	1/0	1/0	1/2	3/5	10/9	83/84
7. Intelligence	1.87/2.00/1.72	1.5 / 1.5 / 1.6	3/2	14/14	26/19	20/20	9/7	28/37
8. Courage, firmness	.42/.49/.32	0.9 / 1.0 / 0.8	1/1	2/0	4/3	8/2	12/13	74/81
9. Wealth	.29/.37/.19	0.9 / 1.0 / 0.7	2/1	2/0	3/2	2/2	7/4	84/91
10. Kindness, softness	.75/.72/.80	1.3 / 1.3 / 1.3	1/1	5/2	5/11	11/9	8/13	70/64

Distribution: 5 – the most important value; 0 – not selected

effect of well-known socializing mechanisms, social maturation. Still, they provide information that is essential from the perspective of educational efforts which should more often include the elements of support by a group of peers and should refer to altruism, especially with reference to young people.

The analysis of the second part of the respondent's answers to questions about personal values important to them shows again that this hierarchy is similar for both students and professionals. However, we can see differences between the two groups as to the frequency of choices. Professionals choose significantly more often good health ($p<.0001$, Cramér's $V=.18$) as well as knowledge and wisdom ($p=.0012$, Cramér's $V=.16$), and kindness ($p=.0021$, Cramér's $V=.16$) as important and very important values. On the other hand, compared to professionals, students valued more love and friendship ($p<.0001$, Cramér's $V=.17$), intelligence ($p=.0487$, Cramér's $V=.12$), courage ($p=.0028$, Cramér's $V=.15$), wealth ($p=.0482$, Cramér's $V=.12$) and good looks ($p=.0252$, Cramér's $V=.13$). From the perspective of education, in order to more effectively influence medical and physiotherapy students it is necessary to refer more frequently to such values as friendship and love, hedonistic needs as well as good looks and intelligence development. In order, however, to have an effective influence on professionals with reference to health, apart from the superior values such as love and friendship a stronger focus should be put on the value of health as a prerequisite for intellectual efficiency as well as joy of life and satisfaction.

Let's try to identify differences existing between all the five surveyed social and professional groups in respect of individual subjective determinants. The differences in self-rated health ($p<.0001$, Cramér's $V=.13$) result mostly from very low self-rated health of nurses and it is a difference statistically significant compared to all the other surveyed groups (from $p<.00001$ for medicine students to $p=.0058$ for physiotherapists). Students do not differ significantly with respect to each other. At the same time, the respondents differ in a similar way in terms of their attitude to health as a personal value ($p<0001$, Cramér's $V=.13$). This time it is the nurses for whom the value of health is significantly higher than for physicians ($p=.0078$), physiotherapy students ($p=.0004$) and medicine students ($p<.0001$). The situation is similar as for the perception of health as a prerequisite for happiness. The surveyed groups differ in this regard ($p=.0001$, Cramér's $V=.14$). Most often such health value is highly important to nurses and they differ here significantly from physiotherapists ($p=.0049$) and physiotherapy students ($p=.0317$). Therefore, nurses are characterized on the one hand by the awareness of limitations or decreasing potential of their own health, visible in low self-rated health, and on the other hand by a higher valuation of health as a prerequisite for happiness. And students, for whom the time of education, youth and independence quite often is the best time of their lives, irrespective of their field of study, made very similar choices regarding the health value and self-rated health.

In the next stage, the analysis focused on self-efficacy in individual health behaviours. The differences in self-efficacy related to all the analysed health behaviours were observed between the surveyed groups in the field of physical activity self-efficacy (p<.0001, η²=.04), nutrition self-efficacy (p=.0019, η²=.02), alcohol self-efficacy (p<.0001, η²=.05) and smoking self-efficacy (p=.0184, η²=.02). Among professionals nurses have physical activity self-efficacy significantly lower compared to physiotherapists (p=.0012) and physicians (p=.0008). Students of physiotherapy and medicine do not differ from each other while their physical activity self-efficacy is significantly higher than that of nurses (p<.0001 for the both groups). Similarly to students, professionals do not differ in their self-rated nutrition self-efficacy. A group least confident in their nutrition self-efficacy among all the respondents includes physiotherapists whose scores are lower than those of both physiotherapy (p=.0118) and medical (p=.0135) students. As for alcohol self-efficacy, physiotherapists had the lowest scores among professionals (p=.0198 compared to physicians, p=.0119 compared to nurses). The difference was also visible among students. Physiotherapy students assessed their ability to cope with the temptation to drink alcohol lower (p=.0012) than medical students. Generally, in all the surveyed groups physiotherapists ranked the lowest in terms of alcohol self-efficacy, also compared to medical (p=.0012) and physiotherapy (p=.0345) students. Professionals differed also in the assessment of their smoking self-efficacy, where nurses had the lowest self-efficacy for ability to cope with the temptation to smoke (p=.0324 compared to physicians). Students had a similar assessment of their self-efficacy. Nurses scored their self-efficacy also significantly lower than physiotherapy students (p=.0254).

The analysis included also differences in the respondents' health locus of control. Such differences between the groups were revealed in all the three distinguished types of health locus of control. Internal Health Locus of Control (p=.0058, η²=.02) did not differentiate the groups of professionals and students. However, it was highest among physiotherapy students and, interestingly, lowest among physiotherapists (p=.0097). Physiotherapy students have also Internal Health Locus of Control significantly higher than nurses (p=.0289). Confidence in own abilities and conviction of independence in deciding about own health is also relatively high among physicians. It may be assumed that as a result of life experience, especially professional experience, this conviction is lower among physiotherapists. The respondents show differences (p=.0035, η²=.02) also in the area of external health control related to authorities (Powerful Others Health Locus of Control). Physiotherapists ranked the lowest and they significantly differ from nurses (p=.0012). In other words, they least trust external authorities when it comes to their own health and, contrary to nurses, are not willing to give them control over their own health. However, they showed the highest scores for Powerful Others Health Locus of Control. Though both professional groups are related to the area of health and disease, they still have quite different profiles with regard to health locus of control. It may be assumed that physiotherapists should be or necessarily have to be independent in their therapeutic activities. However, because they often encounter physicians' ignorance about the health services provided by physiotherapists, they, lack confidence in physicians' and medical authorities' competence. On the other hand, due to their professional relations, especially with physicians, nurses should trust authorities in that regard in order to competently and safely perform their professional duties. It is also a kind of adaptive mechanism to the professional role they fulfill. The third type of control, also external but independent from anyone and anything but fate or chance, namely Chance Health Locus of Control was highest also among nurses (p=.0175, η^2=.02). This professional group is particularly vulnerable to external influences and least confident in their own ability to decide about their own health.

The analysis included also biological determinants (correlates) of health behaviours, such as BMI, waist circumference, WHR, incidence of lifestyle diseases. They are listed in Table 4.14.

One of the basic nutrition indexes, resulting from a particular lifestyle, is BMI. BMI values are age-independent and the same for both sexes. However, BMI may not correspond to the same degree of fatness in different populations, in part due to different body proportions. The average for the respondents is within the norm. Students have BMI significantly lower than professionals (p<.001, Hedges' g=.29) – small effect. Nurses compare unfavorably since their average falls within the overweight category. Around 7% of BMI variance is explained by the membership in the surveyed groups (F(4,760)=13.71, p<.0001, η^2=.07). Similarly, as shown by epidemiological trends, the percentage of overweight people increases with age and this problem affects particularly often nurses, slightly less often physicians and every fifth physiotherapist. It is a particularly important observation in the context of the educational role that the both professional groups should play in the promotion of physical activity and proper nutrition, directly related to this index.

The most recent WHO recommendations indicate significant prediction between waist circumferences/WHR and cardiovascular as well as metabolic diseases (Waist Circumference and *Waist-Hip* Ratio, 2011). In this study we have respondents' statements regarding this issue and the research recorded the highest number of missing answers to that question (up to 30% for individual groups); therefore, we present only approximate trends achieved while being aware of limitations of the material gathered. Nevertheless, similar to the case of BMI, the percentage of higher waist circumferences increases with the age of the respondents. A particularly unfavorable increase can be observed among women, where students have significantly lower scores than professional women (p<.0001, Hedges' g=.76) – large effect, whereas circumferences risky to health are most frequently observed in nurses (27%) (see Fig. 4.21), and the unfavorable WHRs is present in approximately 30% of the respondents.

Table 4.14 Stratification of respondents' biological characteristics

		All	students		professionals			p value[a] effect size	p value[b] effect size
			medical	physiotherapy	physicians	nurses	physiotherapists		
BMI	M ± SD	22.8 ± 4.0	22.1±4.1	22.2±2.9	23.4±3.0	25.1±4.1	22.4±5.1	p<.001 g=.29	p<.001 η^2=.07
Waist (cm)									
	M ± SD	74.7±8.8	75.0±8.1	71.1±6.5	74.9±8.7	80.2±9.2	71.7±7.3	p<.0001 g=.76	p<.0001 η^2=.19
	M ± SD	86.4±11.3	89.0±10.1	86.1±11.6	92.0±9.0	96.7±12.7	96.0±8.1	p=.742 ns	p=.998 ns
Diseases:									
Hypertension	n	57	10	1	19	19	8		
Overweight	n	61	16	12	8	14	11		
Atherosclerosis	n	4	0	0	2	1	1		
Diabetes	n	4	2	2	0	0	0		
CVD	n	25	9	0	7	9	0		
Allergy	n	142	58	54	13	11	6		

a – test t was used for differences between students/professionals and Hedges' g effect size
b – one-way ANOVA was used for differences between all groups and eta squared effect size (η^2)

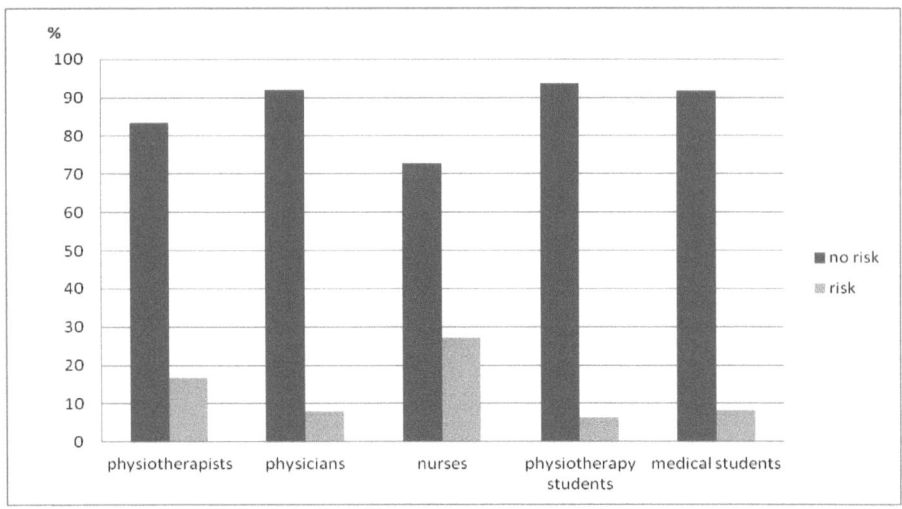

Figure 4.21 Risky waist circumferences (percentages of respondents)

According to respondents' statements only a few have been diagnosed as having one of the lifestyle diseases. Allergy is the most frequent chronic disease reported by the respondents. When we look at the interaction between the frequency of incidence of particular diseases and BMI, we can see that the co-occurrence of overweight and hypertension is more often declared by overweight persons whereas CVDs by persons with normal BMI (p<.00001). Persons who declared that they suffered from any particular lifestyle related disease (hypertension, CVD, atherosclerosis) either failed to provide information on their waist circumferences or had them normal. It was only obesity that was reported more often by persons with dangerously higher waist circumferences or WHRs. This fact may suggest that some remedial actions were already taken, the etiology of the mentioned diseases is different.

4.4 Personal and Social Determinants of Health Behaviour

The second stage of the analysis included the search for relationships between individual determinants (psychosocial and biological), social determinants and health behaviour. The following subjective health determinants were taken into account in the analysis: health locus of control, health-specific self-efficacy, place of health in the hierarchy of values, health as a prerequisite for happiness, self-rated health, BMI as well as social health determinants such as stage of professional career and type of education. The same analysis procedure was employed with regard to each of the analysed behaviours. There were two models distinguished in the procedure. In order to assess the relationship between each of the behaviours and each independent variable, first we conducted a logistic regression analysis with each of the behaviours as the dependent variable and each variable as the independent one. This model (Model I) estimated the potential risk of behaviour adverse to health with reference to all the analysed independent (subject and social) variables. Then, all factors were entered in a logistic regression model with backward elimination of variable selection. As a result, the final model (Model II) was estimated, which consists of significant variables only.

4.4.1 Physical Activity

Physical activity is one of those behavioural factors the decline of which has been observed in the developed countries for years. In this chapter the assessment was made of relationships between subject variables (health locus of control measured by Multidementional Health Locus fo Control Scale – MHLC, physical activity self-efficacy – PA SE, place of health in the hierarchy of values, health as a prerequisite for happiness, self-rated health, BMI) as well as social variables (stage of professional career and type of education) and the level of physical activity. Physical activity was analysed as a dichotomous measure. Behaviour beneficial to health was considered to be the one in which health recommendations are implemented within that scope (high level in the IPAQ questionnaire). The other behaviours were found to be adverse. Models of one- and multi-dimensional logistic regression were estimated (Tab. 4.15). Model I contains the results of estimation of the risk of low (insufficient for health) physical activity with reference to all the analysed subject and social variables. Model II presents the final determination model resulting from multiple backward logistic regression for p<.05.

Table 4.15 Risk factors associated with low PA – odds ratio from logistic regression

Factors		MODEL I Physical activity		MODEL II Physical activity		
		OR (95% CI[b])	p value	Beta	OR (95% CI)	p value
PA SE	High	ref.				
	Medium	3.88 (2.56-5.87)	.000	0.40	1.49 (1.17-1.90)	.001
	Low	4.14 (2.74-6.24)	.000	0.43	1.53 (1.20-1.95)	.001
MHCL Internal (ref.[a] high)		1.55 (1.14-2.10)	.005			
MHCL Powerful (ref. high)		0.81 (0.59-1.10)	.170			
MHCL Chance (ref. high)		0.54 (0.40-0.74)	.000	0.27	0.77 (0.65-0.91)	.003

Table 4.15 Risk factors associated with low PA – odds ratio from logistic regression _{continued}

Factors		MODEL I Physical activity			MODEL II Physical activity	
		OR (95% CI[b])	p value	Beta	OR (95% CI)	p value
HEALTH as a value	5 the most important	ref.				
	4	1.04 (0.70-1.54)	.851			
	3	1.19 (0.68-2.09)	.540			
	2	1.54 (0.88-2.69)	.127			
	1 the least important	1.12 (0.57-2.23)	.736			
	0 not chosen	1.45 (0.81-2.61)	.214			
HEALTH as a happiness	5 the most important	ref.				
	4	1.25 (0.84-1.88)	.277			
	3	1.22 (0.77-1.94)	.405			
	2	0.78 (0.45-1.36)	.382			
	1 the least important	0.77 (0.40-1.45)	.417			
	0 not chosen	1.57 (0.84-2.93)	.158			
Self-rated Health	very good	ref.				
	good	2.41 (1.63-3.57)	.000	0.33	1.39 (0.90-2.13)	.134
	moderate	3.32 (1.96-5.62)	.000	0.34	1.40 (0.85-2.31)	.185
	bad or very bad	2.16 (0.55-8.38)	.267	0.15	0.86 (0.29-2.60)	.792
BMI	normal weight I	ref.				
	underweight	2.22 (1.10-4.47)	.026	0.39	1.48 (0.83-2.65)	.188
	normal weight II	1.69 (1.11-2.58)	.015	0.20	1.22 (0.84-1.78)	.295
	overweight	1.59 (1.08-2.35)	.019	0.24	0.79 (0.54-1.14)	.208
Career Stage	student	ref.				
	professional	1.44 (1.06-1.95)	.021			
Groups	medical st.	ref.				
	physiotherapy st.	0.56 (0.37-0.85)	.007	0.70	0.50 (0.36-0.69)	.000
	nurse	1.49 (0.90-2.45)	.122	0.24	1.27 (0.84-1.92)	.250
	physiotherapist	0.74 (0.46-1.18)	.202	0.34	0.71 (0.50-1.02)	.065
	physician	1.33 (0.81-2.20)	.265	0.62	1.85 (1.22-2.80)	.004

a – ref: reference group; b – CI: Confidence interval

Self-efficacy is a well-known predictor of health behaviours. One might have expected that its role would be strong in the analysed relationships. Persons with an average level of this competence are at almost four times greater risk of being physically inactive whereas the risk is more than four times greater for persons having a low self-efficacy level. Out of the three types of Health Locus of Control only two – Internal Control and Chance Control – proved to be significantly related to the risk of low physical activity but in different ways. Persons with a low sense of internal control are 55% more at risk of sedentary behaviour whereas a low sense of control over one's health, i.e. reluctance to leave health choices to chance or fate reduces this risk to 46%. The valuing of health as both an important personal value and a prerequisite for happiness does not differentiate respondents in terms of their physical activity. On the other hand, self-rated health is visibly related to the level of the respondents' physical activity. The lower the respondents rated their health the greater was the risk of being physically inactive (two or three times). Similarly, the risk was higher as the body weight increased and even more (more than two times) when the body weight was below the norm. Social factors related to education and career stage also differentiated the respondent's behaviours. In the case of professionals the risk of no activity increases by 44% whereas based on the comparison of all the analysed social and professional groups the risk of being insufficiently physically active was lowest for physiotherapy students.

In the next stage (Model II) we sought multidimensional prediction of sedentary behaviours, taking all the aforementioned variables into consideration. Within 7 steps the best-fitting model was obtained, with 5 out of all the distinguished factors taken into account: physical activity self-efficacy, Chance Health Locus of Control, Self-rate Health, BMI and Groups. The following can be considered as factors predisposing to low physical activity: declining self-rated health, underweight, average or low sense of physical activity self-efficacy, high sense of control over our health by fate or chance. Physiotherapy education seems to be a particularly protecting factor whereas being a physician significantly increases the risk of sedentary behaviours.

4.4.2 Nutrition

Adverse nutrition behaviours are one of the essential risk factors for chronic diseases and diseases of civilization. People who do not put any effort or do not find any pleasure in proper nutrition most often excuse themselves by citing a lack of time, so typical of all the analysed respondent groups. Another factor related to nutrition behaviours is specialist knowledge (nutrition literacy). The surveyed professional groups should form the first front line group for educational activities in this area. Medical and physiotherapy studies are supposed to prepare also for that role; however, the effects of this education in the form of preferred nutrition models may give rise to considerable reservations which are further analysed in this chapter.

The analysis procedure used was the same as for physical activity determinants. The adverse pattern of behaviours was determined in two ways. First, by taking into account all the 12 studied behaviours (NI12), indicating both quantity and frequency of consumption of individual products and meals and by developing sten norms for them in the analysed group. The analysis of the results obtained can be found in Table 16. In the logistic modeling the adverse pattern of behaviour was assumed to be values corresponding to 1 sten (low values), the value of two subsequent ones were treated jointly. The other method used was based on the most important dietary risk factors: consumption of complex carbohydrates, vegetables and fruits (NI3). Each of these behaviours was described as: beneficial (3 points) – everyday consumption of the aforementioned products, moderately beneficial (2 points) – several times a week, adverse (1 point) – more rarely than several times a week (details see: section Study Design). On that basis, a beneficial pattern was developed and it assumed the possibility of moderate departure from one behaviour at maximum, i.e. obtaining at least 8 points. The lowest score indicated the adverse pattern of nutrition behaviours.

The results of the prediction of the nutrition behaviour pattern adverse to health (NI12 and NI3) are presented in Model I whereas Model II shows the results of multiple backward logistic regression.

Table 4.16 Risk factors associated with unhealthy nutrition habits NI12.

Factors		MODEL I NI12		MODEL II NI12		
		OR (95% CI[b])	p value	Beta	OR (95% CI)	p value
NI12 SE	High	ref.				
	Medium	1.29 (0.88-1.91)	.196	0.12	1.13 (0.88-1.44)	.333
	Low	1.89 (1.29-2.79)	.001	0.25	1.28 (0.99-1.66)	.056
MHCL Internal (ref.[a] high)		1.09 (0.81-1.47)	.566			
MHCL Powerful (ref. high)		0.71 (0.53-0.96)	.026			
MHCL Chance (ref. high)		0.56 (0.41-0.76)	.000			
HEALTH as a value	5 the most important	ref.				
	4	1.12 (0.76-1.66)	.554			
	3	1.40 (0.80-2.46)	.236			
	2	1.09 (0.62-1.91)	.772			
	1 the least important	0.83 (0.41-1.68)	.610			
	0 not chosen	2.19 (1.27-3.77)	.005			

_{continued}**Table 4.16** Risk factors associated with unhealthy nutrition habits NI12.

Factors		MODEL I NI12			MODEL II NI12	
		OR (95% CI[b])	p value	Beta	OR (95% CI)	p value
HEALTH as a happiness	5 the most important	ref.				
	4	0.74 (0.44-1.11)	.143			
	3	1.15 (0,73-1.80)	.548			
	2	1.02 (0.61-1.71)	.945			
	1 the least important	0.83 (0.44-1.57)	.567			
	0 not chosen	1.57 (0.88-2.79)	.124			
Self-rated Health	very good	ref.				
	good	2.36 (1.59-3.49)	.000	0.00	1.00 (0.65-1,54)	.992
	moderate	3.43 (2.03-5.78)	.000	0.34	1.41 (0.83-2.38)	.203
	bad or very bad	3.29 (0.96-11.33)	.059	0.22	1.24 (0.41-3.75)	.703
BMI	normal weight I	ref.				
	underweight	1.26 (0.66-2.42)	.487	0.29	1.34 (0.76-2.36)	.315
	normal weight II	0.54 (0.34-0.87)	.012	-0.61	0.54 (0.36-0.83)	.004
	overweight	1.89 (1.32-2.72)	.001	0.50	1.65 (1.14-2.38)	.008
Career Stage	student	ref.				
	professional	0.68 (0.50-0.91)	.011			
Groups	medical st.	ref.				
	physiotherapy st.	1.61 (1.09-2.39)	.018	0.66	1.93 (1.40-2.65)	.000
	nurse	1.22 (0.76-1.96)	.403	-0.20	0.82 (0.54-1.24)	.343
	physiotherapist	0.61 (0.37-1.01)	.057	-0.44	0.65 (0.43-0.98)	.038
	physician	0.81 (0.49-1.34)	.417	-0.12	0.89 (0.57-1.39)	.607

a – ref: reference group; b – CI: Confidence interval

Similar to physical activity, self-efficacy as to how prepare healthful foods is related to more beneficial nutrition behaviours. Persons with low self-efficacy in that area are almost twice as likely to have improper diet. As for the analysed types of Health Locus of Control, Others Control and Chance Control proved to be significantly differentiating the risk of adverse behaviours. Persons with a low sense of external control, both related to authorities and to chance or fate are 29% and 44%, respectively, less likely to follow an unhealthy diet. The tendency for giving control over one's own health to external factors such as physicians, specialists or fate, God and chance contributes to more frequent abandonment of efforts made by the respondents to follow a diet more beneficial to health.

The position of health in the system of values and its appreciation in the context of personal happiness are not factors differentiating behaviours of the respondents. However, the worse the respondents rated their health the more likely they were to have adverse behaviours, with the risk higher more than three times for the poor and bad rates. On the other hand, unsurprisingly, the risk of adverse nutrition behaviours increased by almost 90% can be observed in overweight persons. While analyzing differences between the surveyed social and professional groups, we can see that the fact of being a student increases that risk whereas the risk is lower in the case of physiotherapists and physicians by almost 40% and 20%, respectively, compared to medical students.

Model II presents the results of multidimensional prediction of nutrition behaviours adverse to health, taking all the aforementioned variables into consideration. In the final model obtained in 8 steps 4 factors were included, namely: nutrition self-efficacy, BMI, Self-rated Health, Groups. Factors particularly protecting against adverse nutrition behaviours seem to include high self-efficacy in dealing with the organization of proper nutrition, low sense of external control as well as working as physiotherapist or physician.

Table. 4.17 Risk factors associated with unhealthy nutrition habits NI3

Factors		MODEL I NI3			MODEL II NI3	
		OR (95% CI[b])	p value	Beta	OR (95% CI)	p value
NI3 SE	High	ref.				
	Medium	1.85 (1.30-2.50)	.001	0.23	1.26 (0.99-1.59)	.060
	Low	2.35 (1.63-3.39)	.000	0.60	1.82 (1.41-2.34)	.000
MHCL Internal (ref.[a] high)		1.06 (0.80-1.41)	.678			
MHCL Powerful (ref. high)		0.91 (0.69-1.22)	.539	-0.18	0.83 (0.70-0.99)	.041
MHCL Chance (ref. high)		0.76 (0.57-1.01)	.056			
HEALTH as a value	5 the most important	ref.				
	4	0.98 (0.68-1.41)	.915			
	3	0.98 (0.57-1.68)	.942			
	2	1.02 (0.60-1.73)	.939			
	1 the least important	1.63 (0.84-3.15)	.149			
	0 not chosen	1.15 (0.67-1.96)	.621			

continued**Table. 4.17** Risk factors associated with unhealthy nutrition habits NI3

Factors		MODEL I NI3			MODEL II NI3	
		OR (95% CI[b])	p value	Beta	OR (95% CI)	p value
HEALTH as a happiness	5 the most important	ref.				
	4	0.88 (0.60-1.28)	.500			
	3	0.94 (0.61-1.46)	.788			
	2	0.76 (0.46-1.24)	.269			
	1 the least important	0.82 (0.45-1.47)	.498			
	0 not chosen	1.28 (0.71-2.31)	.403			
Self-rated Health	very good	ref.				
	good	1.31 (0.94-1.83)	.108			
	moderate	1.44 (0.88-2.34)	.146			
	bad or very bad	0.53 (0.15-1.88)	.328			
BMI	normal weight I	ref.				
	underweight	0.82 (0.44-1.53)	.530	-0.40	0.67 (0.38-1.19)	.172
	normal weight II	0.76 (0.51-1.12)	.168	0.02	1.02 (0.70-1.48)	.938
	overweight	1.46 (1.01-2.10)	.045	0.55	1.73 (1.18-2.54)	.005
Career Stage	student	ref.				
	professional	0.44 (0.33-0.59)	.000			
Groups	medical st.	ref.				
	physiotherapy st.	1.83 (1.22-2.76)	.004	0.98	2.68 (1.89-3.78)	.000
	nurse	0.91 (0.58-1.44)	.702	-0.06	0.94 (0.63-1.40)	.752
	physiotherapist	0.47 (0.30-0.73)	.001	-0.49	0.61 (0.43-0.88)	.008
	physician	0.47 (0.30-0.75)	.001	-0.58	0.56 (0.38-0.84)	.005

a – ref: reference group; b – CI: Confidence interval

A prediction analysis was made for NI3 based on the three most important diet elements: everyday consumption of complex carbohydrates, vegetables and fruits. Factors related to the greatest risk of adverse nutrition are similar to those for NI12. Persons with moderate or low self-efficacy are almost twice or over twice, respectively, as likely to have improper diet. Persons with a low sense of external control related to chance or fate are 24% less likely to follow an unhealthy diet. The valuation of health does not differentiate nutrition behaviours. Similarly, health self-rating does not differentiate the respondents in terms of risk of low consumption of vegetables, fruits and complex carbohydrates but it differentiates them in terms of NI12. The observation of the risk of adverse nutrition behaviours increased by 46% in overweight persons is not surprising. The risk of insufficient consumption of vegetables, fruits and complex carbohydrates occurs more often in students than in professionals whereas in the case of physiotherapists and physicians it is lower by more than 50% compared to medical students.

Model II presents the result of multidimensional prediction of nutrition behaviours adverse to health, taking all the aforementioned variables into consideration. In the final model obtained in 8 steps 4 factors were included, namely: nutrition self-efficacy, Powerful Others Health Locus of Control, BMI, Groups. Factors particularly protecting against adverse nutrition behaviours seem to include high self-efficacy in dealing with the organization of proper nutrition, low sense of external control as well as working as physiotherapist or physician.

4.4.3 Smoking

Smoking is one of the most important risk factors for the diseases of civilization, including in particular tumors and diseases of circulatory and respiratory system. The combined forces of medicine, politics, governmental and non-governmental organizations have gone to war against this terrible addiction. As a result, for years we have observed a downward trend in the number of smokers and various statutory solutions contribute to this trend. Unfortunately, medical circles in Poland do not set a good example in this regard, especially if we look at certain specializations, e.g. surgeons. The sight of a smoking physician or even a smoking physician seeing patients is still not so rare. A ban on smoking in public places introduced in Poland in November 2010 has definitely improved the situation. We can observe alarming statistics among young people where the percentage of smokers is even growing in certain circles; therefore, both monitoring and an attempt to define new remedies are required. A procedure identical to the one used for physical activity and nutrition was employed also for the analysis of determinants of smoking among the respondents.

The analysis was performed with reference to the risk of smoking at any time, i.e. being both a current smoker and an ex-smoker were considered to be a risky behaviour. The results of smoking prediction are presented in Model I whereas Model II gives the results of multiple backward logistic regression (Tab. 4.18).

It is no surprise that people overcoming various temptations and obstacles in the process of quitting smoking or not taking up smoking are definitely less exposed to this risk. The risk increases strongly when this confidence is missing, from more than 5 times in persons with moderate self-efficacy to more than 50 times in persons with low self-efficacy in this regard. It is by far the most significant competence out of those analysed in the context of smoking. As for Health Locus of Control, Internal Control and Powerful Others Control differentiated the behaviours in a similar way. The risk of succumbing to addiction increases by almost 40% when the respondents have a low sense of Internal Control, i.e. they do not rely on their own judgments and are not sure about their resolutions related to health. Also people with a low sense

Table 4.18 Risk factors associated with smoking

Factors		MODEL I Smoking			MODEL II Smoking	
		OR (95% CI[b])	p value	Beta	OR (95% CI)	p value
Smoking SE	High	ref.				
	Medium	5.30 (3.14-8.94)	.000	-0.16	0.85 (0.58-1.26)	.421
	Low	56.04 (33.72-93.11)	.000	2.11	8.24 (5.63-12.07)	.000
MHCL Internal (ref.[a] high)		1.38 (1.01-1.89)	.042			
MHCL Powerful (ref. high)		1.47 (1.07-2.02)	.016			
MHCL Chance (ref. high)		1.11 (0.82-1.52)	.496			
HEALTH as a value	5 the most important	ref.				
	4	0.85 (0.57-1.26)	.415			
	3	0.62 (0.32-1.17)	.141			
	2	1.05 (0.59-1.87)	.867			
	1 the least important	1.67 (0.87-3.19)	.121			
	0 not chosen	1.80 (1.04-3.13)	.037			
HEALTH as a happiness	5 the most important	ref.				
	4	1.00 (0.66-1.53)	.991			
	3	1.79 (1.13-2.84)	.013			
	2	0.81 (0.45-1.45)	.474			
	1 the least important	0.90 (0.46-1.77)	.766			
	0 not chosen	1.42 (0.77-2.61)	.257			
Self-rated Health	very good	ref.				
	good	1.93 (1.28-2.91)	.002			
	moderate	4.64 (2.72-7.92)	.000			
	bad or very bad	5.57 (1.61-19.24)	.007			
BMI		1.13 (1.08-1.18)	.000	0.12	1.13 (1.06-1.21)	.000
Career Stage Groups	student	ref.				
	professional	2.16 (1.57-2.96)	.000			
	medical st.	ref.				
	physiotherapy st.	0.75 (0.47-1.19)	.222	-0.64	0.53 (0.33-0.85)	.009
	nurse	2.28 (1.41-3.70)	.001	0.06	1.07 (0.63-1.81)	.816
	physiotherapist	1.95 (1.22-3.14)	.006	0.68	1.96 (1.21-3.20)	.007
	physician	1.48 (0.90-2.45)	.123	0.59	1.80 (1.07-3.01)	.026

a – ref: reference group; b – CI: Confidence interval

of Powerful Others Control are nearly 50% more likely to smoke. The reluctance to become influenced by authorities that may be associated with those informing about dangers arising from smoking as well as the fact of not accepting information already publicly available on the dangers of smoking may be a mechanism that facilitates succumbing to temptation or otherwise hinder the fight against addiction. However, the awareness of health damage related to smoking can be observed among the students and professionals participating in the study. The risk of smoking clearly increases along with the decrease in Self-rated Health (from two to five times). A particular increase can be observed among those rating their health as moderate or bad and very bad. Due to incomplete categories in some classes, BMI was treated as continuous variable in the model. The higher the index the more likely a person is to smoke. While analyzing differences in the risk of smoking in the surveyed groups we can observe that the risk faced by professionals is two times higher and nurses compare particularly unfavorably (risk greater more than two times) in a detailed analysis of all the distinguished groups.

Model II presents the result of backward logistic regression analysis. In the final model obtained in 9 steps three factors were included, namely: smoking self-efficacy, BMI and Career Stage. The factors particularly predisposing to a higher risk of smoking include: low sense of self-efficacy in dealing with the temptation to smoke, higher BMI and taking up a professional job.

4.4.4 Alcohol Consumption

Poland is quite unequivocally associated with a particular alcohol use pattern, the so-called eastern pattern, still typical of Russia or post-communist countries, i.e. the consumption of mainly high-proof alcohols and in large quantities. This model has been quite strongly evolving though it is still present or even popular in some social circles. Currently, the problem of alcohol abuse more and more often concerns the elite, including medical circles, and not only the poor from the dregs of society. It is extremely difficult to get real answers from such aware and educated groups as those included in this study. Nevertheless, with a probable underestimation of the problem in mind, determinants of alcohol consumption in the groups of respondents are presented below. The employed procedure was analogous to that described in the preceding chapters: Model I – the results of a logistic regression analysis, Model II – the results of a backward stepwise logistic regression analysis (Tab. 4.19).

Just like in the case of the other addictions, a low sense of self-efficacy is associated with more than five times greater risk of an adverse behaviour pattern related to alcohol consumption. As for Health Locus of Control, a low belief in Powerful Others Control reduces the risk of adverse behaviours by 28% whereas a low belief in Change Control increases it by more than 50%. In other words, persons not submitting to influences of others on their own health are less likely to face the risk of alcohol consumption adverse to health, similarly to those who count on luck or chance in maintaining good health. Distinct differences emerged between the surveyed groups. Professionals

Table 4.19 Risk factors associated with alcohol consumption

Factors		MODEL I Alcohol			MODEL II Alcohol	
		OR (95% CI[b])	p value	Beta	OR (95% CI)	p value
Alcohol SE	High	ref.				
	Medium	3.77 (2.04-6.97)	.000	0.50	1.65 (1.12-2.45)	.012
	Low	5.49 (3.09-9.74)	.000	0.57	1.77 (1.25-2.50)	.001
MHCL Internal (ref.[a] high)		1.08 (0.78-1.48)	.650	0.29	1.34 (1.02-1,75)	.034
MHCL Powerful (ref. high)		0.72 (0.52-0.99)	.041	-0.39	0.68 (0.52-0.89)	.004
MHCL Chance (ref. high)		1.54 (1.11-2.12)	.009	0.42	1.52 (1.16-2.00)	.003
HEALTH as a value	5 the most important	ref.				
	4	0.73 (0.48-1.10)	.130			
	3	1.05 (0.58-1.89)	.870			
	2	1.17 (0.65-2.09)	.608			
	1 the least important	1.86 (0.98-3.55)	.059			
	0 not chosen	1.10 (0.61-1.96)	.753			
HEALTH as a happiness	5 the most important	ref.				
	4	0.78 (0.51-1.20)	.263			
	3	0.95 (0.59-1.54)	.838			
	2	0.90 (0.51-1.58)	.716			
	1 the least important	1.08 (0.57-2.04)	.824			
	0 not chosen	1.47 (0.80-2.69)	.214			
Self-rated Health	very good	ref.				
	good	1.18 (0.81-1.72)	.393			
	moderate	1.21 (0.71-2.09)	.484			
	bad or very bad	0.65 (0.14-3.08)	.583			
BMI	normal weight I	ref.				
	underweight	1.66 (0.87-3.17)	.125			
	normal weight II	1.11 (0.72-1.72)	.630			
	over weight	0.74 (0.49-1.13)	.164			
Career Stage Groups	student	ref.				
	professional	0.51 (0.36-0.71)	.000			
	medical st.	ref.				
	physiotherapy st.	0.62 (0.41-0.93)	.020			
	nurse	0.16 (0.08-0.32)	.000			
	physiotherapist	0.69 (0.43-1.10)	.120			
	physician	0.41 (0.24-0.70)	.001			

a – ref: reference group; b – CI: Confidence interval

are about half as likely to drink alcohol in a risky manner as students. Moreover, if we look at the groups in detail, it appears that the risk of too excessive consumption of alcohol in almost all the surveyed social and professional groups is from 40% to 80% lower than in the case of medical students.

Model II presents the result of backward logistic regression analysis. In the final model obtained in 8 steps four factors were included, namely: Chance Health Locus of Control, Powerful Others Health Locus of Control, Internal Health Locus of Control and alcohol self-efficacy. The factors protecting against alcohol use adverse to health include: high sense of self-efficacy, high sense of Chance Control and Internal Control as well as low sense of Powerful Others Control.

4.5 Mediation of Health Behaviours

In the third stage of the analysis a question was posed about the mediator role of selected variables in taking up the analysed health behaviours. The selection and classification of variables were made taking the strength and stability of the studied psychological constructs defined as determinants of health behaviours into account. The analysis relied on Wiefferink et al. (2006) clustering of health behaviours and their determinants, based on the Theory of Triadic Influence (TTI) (Flay & Petraitis, 1994). This integrative theory combines determinants of health behaviours at different levels (i.e. proximal, distal, ultimate) but also determinants of different types (i.e. intrapersonal and interpersonal). This analysis did not include any ultimate-level variables. Only social economic status in self-perception of respondents is known from this level. However, the surveyed group is quite homogenous in many respects since it includes medical service workers educated in the same – biomedical – field and students preparing to work in similar jobs. The analysis included the following distal level variables: in the biology/personality stream – health locus of control; in the culture stream – health place in the personal values system and health place as a symbol of personal happiness. The analysis included also the following proximal level variables: in the biology/personality stream: health-specific self-efficacy. On that basis, the models verified by mediation analysis were developed. Health-specific self-efficacy was considered to be the main mediator variable for the analysed behaviours.

In the study dependency hypotheses were verified according to the mediation analysis described in the section on statistical analysis. First, a relationship was sought between the independent variable (from the group of distal determinants) and the mediator variable (from proximal or distal determinants). The correlation coefficients for this relationship were defined as path "a" value. If the value proved to be insignificant, and as a result, did not allow confirming the mediation hypothesis, such results were not presented in the paper. However, if a significant value of the coefficient of path "a" was obtained, the null hypothesis of indirect effect was tested according to the assumptions described in the section Statistical Analysis. The results of the completed analyses are presented in Table 4.20. They are described for individual health behaviour below.

4.5.1 Physical Activity

First, a mediator role of physical activity self-efficacy was examined in the relationship between health valuation as a symbol of happiness or as a personal value and physical activity (PA). The self-efficacy does not play a mediator role in this relationship. Next, a mediator role was examined in the relationship between Health Locus of Control and the level of physical activity. Physical activity self-efficacy plays such a role in the relationship between Internal Health Locus of Control and physical activity. The indirect effect was estimated at .07 (the medium size effect). The 95% confidence interval did not include 0 (C.I.: .06-.10), indicating that the proposed mediation was significant. People with high Internal Health Locus of Control have higher physical activity self-efficacy which affects the level of physical activity. Also Chance Health Locus of Control mediates this relationship. The indirect effect was estimated at -.04 (C.I.: (-.06- (-.01)) – the small size effect. People with a low Chance Health Locus of Control have higher physical activity self-efficacy which affects the level of physical activity. No such correlation was found for Powerful Others Health Locus of Control. Next, a mediator role of individual types of health locus of control was examined for the relationship between the valuation of health as a symbol of happiness or as a personal value and physical activity. Internal Health Locus of Control plays a mediator role for the relationship between the valuation of health as a symbol of happiness and physical activity. The indirect effect was estimated at .02 (C.I: .003-.03) – the small size effect. People who valuated health as an important symbol of happiness have more likely high Internal Health Locus of Control which affects physical activity.

4.5.2 Nutrition

Just like in the case of physical activity, nutrition self-efficacy does not mediate the relationship between the valuation of health as a symbol of happiness or as a personal value and nutrition index taking all the twelve studied nutrition elements into account (NI12). However, nutrition self-efficacy plays a mediator role in the relationship between health locus of control and nutrition – NI12. It is true for Internal Health Locus of Control – the indirect effect was estimated at .05 (C.I.: .03-.08), Chance Health Locus of Control – the indirect effect was estimated at -.03 (C.I.: -.05-(-01)) and Powerful Others Health Locus of Control – the indirect effect was estimated at -.02 (C.I.: -.04-(-.001)). All observed effects are rather small. People with high Internal Health Locus of Control and with low Chance Health Locus of Control or a low Powerful Others Health Locus of Control have more often higher nutritional self-efficacy what affect their dietary habits. Next, a mediator role of individual types of health locus of control was examined in the relationship between the valuation of health as a symbol of happiness or as a personal value and nutrition (NI12). Only Internal Health Locus of Control plays a mediator role for the relationship between the valuation of health as a symbol of happiness and nutrition. The indirect effect was estimated at .01 (C.I.: .001-.02) – small effect. People who value health as a condition of their happiness have more likely high Internal Health Locus of Control what affect physical activity.

For NI3, being an index based on three important diet elements: the consumption of vegetables, fruits and complex carbohydrates, the mediation models similar to those for NI12 were obtained. Nutrition self-efficacy plays this role in the relationship between Internal Health Locus of Control – the indirect effect was estimated at .05 (C.I.: .03-.08), Chance Health Locus of Control – the indirect effect was estimated at -.02 (C.I.: -.04-(-.009)) and Powerful Others Health Locus of Control – the indirect effect was estimated at -.02 (C.I.: -.03-(-.0003)) and nutrition NI3. All observed effects are rather small. People with high Internal Health Locus of Control and with low Chance Health Locus of Control or a low Powerful Others Health Locus of Control have more often higher nutritional self-efficacy what affect dietary habits.

4.5.3 Smoking

Smoking is a categorical variable and therefore, the mediation analysis was performed for dichotomous dependent variables whereas smoking was classified in two categories: a never-smoker and a smoker or ex-smoker. Smoking self-efficacy plays a mediator role in the relationship between the valuation of health as a personal value and smoking – the indirect effect was estimated at .20 (C.I.: .05-.37), as well as in the relationship between Internal Health Locus of Control and smoking - the indirect effect was estimated at .22 (C.I.: .07-.37). These effects are rather large. People who have valued health high or who have high Internal Health Locus of Control have more likely high smoking self-efficacy which effects smoking status. On the other hand, Internal Health Locus of Control (indirect effect: .02 (C.I.: .002-.05)) and Powerful Others Health Locus of Control (indirect effect: .02 (C.I.: .0002-.04) play a mediator role in the relationship between the valuation of health as a symbol of happiness and smoking – small effects. People who have valued health as a symbol of happiness have more likely high Internal Health Locus of Control and they have more likely high Powerful Others Health Locus of Control what effects smoking.

4.5.4 Alcohol Consumption

The consumption of alcohol is a categorical variable and therefore, similar to smoking, it was classified as a dichotomous variable: moderately or less drinking and heavy and binge drinking. Neither alcohol self-efficacy or health locus of control plays a mediator role in the analysed relationships with the level of alcohol consumption.

Table 4.20 Direct, indirect and total effect on health behaviours

Variables			Effects		
Independent	Mediating	Dependent	Direct	Indirect	Total
Internal HLOC	PA SE	PA	.10**	.07 (.06-.10)	.16***
Chance HLOC	PA SE	PA	-.08*	-.04 (-.06-(-.01))	-.11**
Health as happiness	Internal HLOC	PA	.002	.02 (.003-.03)	.02
Internal HLOC	nutrition SE	NI12	.04	.05 (.03-.08)	.09*
Chance HLOC	nutrition SE	NI12	-.09*	-.03 (-.05-(-01))	-.11**
Powerful HLOC	nutrition SE	NI12	.001	-.02 (-.04-(-.001))	-.02
Health as happiness	Internal HLOC	NI12	.02	.01 (.001-.02)	.02
Internal HLOC	nutrition SE	NI3	-.02	.05 (.03-.08)	.03
Chance HLOC	nutrition SE	NI3	-.06	-.02 (-.04-(-.009))	-.09*
Powerful HLOC	nutrition SE	NI3	-.001	-.02 (-.03-(-.0003))	-.02
Health as value	smoking SE	smoking	.09	.20 (.05-.37)	.20**
Internal HLOC	smoking SE	smoking	.001	.22 (.07-.37)	.18*
Health as happiness	Internal HLOC	smoking	.04	.02 (.002-.05)	.06
Health as happiness	Powerful HLOC	smoking	.05	.01 (.0002-.04)	.06

*p<.05, **p<.01, ***p<.001

5 Current and Future Health Professionals as "Role Models" for Patients (Clients) – Implications for the Health Promotion Programme

Health behaviours are an important topic of study for modern public health. They are the main factors contributing to lifestyle diseases which, as diseases of a chronic character, effectively reduce the quality of life and are the leading causes of death among residents of developed countries. Health professionals are perceived as individuals who are competent to give advice and support patients (customers) in overcoming health compromising behaviours and adopting health – promoting ones. They enjoy the considerable social trust, particularly in the field of fighting diseases. But when it comes to help in changing lifestyle, the matter is not so obvious (Hawe et al., 2010).

In Poland, as in many other countries, health professionals enjoy a high level of social trust and medical studies are considered among the most prestigious academic disciplines. However, this recognition is not equal among all the professionals. Clearly, physicians are considered the most prestigious profession. In contrast, even though nurses and physiotherapists also follow higher education they are referred to as medical support personnel. This type of gradation results from professional competence determined by the rules of law and is also reflected in the size of the public trust or its determinant from patients.

Apart from pedagogical and social skills or professional knowledge, medical personnel lifestyle can affect the image of a person's competence. Most probably, smoking, obese physicians or nurses will not be credible while giving advice concerning risk factors associated with lifestyle. If a specialist is not strong and determined enough to follow the guidelines, it is difficult for the patient to be convinced of them (Abramson, Stein, Schaufele, Frates, & Rogan, 2000; Frank, Bhat, & Elon, 2003). Therefore, this study analysed health behaviours of the current and future medical staff to assess their potential for educational activities related to health.

5.1 Physical Activity

When comparing the research results with those from the published literature, different methodology for assessing physical activity presented in the available EU reports or studies should be taken into consideration. As a result, direct comparisons are restricted and have an indicative character. Physical activity of the respondents decreases with age and significantly differentiates students and professionals; this is the well-documented direction of changes in physical activity (Sport and Physical Activity, 2010; Troiano, Berrigan, Dodd, Masse, Tilert, & McDowell, 2008). Physical activity of students is higher than that of professionals, but based on the trend in lifelong physical activity we can expect that it will probably decrease after graduation. Similarly, the physiotherapist profession distinguished itself by increased physical activity both during study and professional work. Such results could have been expected and the differences are already noticeable at the level of studies (Hops et al., 2009). This profession requires higher physical fitness and has been recently studied mainly at universities of physical education which are associated with exercise, activity and physical fitness.

However, another type of observation is important, namely the one associated with physical activity taken up by the current and future medical staff. Fewer than 40% of the respondents (physicians and nurses) engage in physical activity intensely enough to develop healthy lifestyles. The findings are similar to the studies on physicians in Poland (Gacek, 2011). Overall in students, 48% of medical students and more than 60% of physiotherapy students show satisfactory frequency of physical activity. Another study indicates that 40% of the adult population in Poland regularly undertake physical activity (Aktywność fizyczna Polaków, 2013). Higher education generally promotes physical activity (Cotter & Lachman, 2010; Dowda, Ainsworth, Saunders, & Riner, 2003) though it's not always so obvious, particularly in transition countries such as Poland. As a result, the percentage values obtained for physically active Poles with higher education vary in different studies. The medical community, especially physicians, belong to the occupational group that has acquired opportunities for rapid economic development associated with the necessity for additional workload and employment. At the same time, physical activity of this occupational group is mainly associated with leisure time. Consequently, physicians have fewer opportunities to catch up on a backlog and undertake a recommended level of daily physical activity. Similarly we have observed the low physical activity of physicians in Europe (Pardo, 2012) and osteotherapists in the United States (McNerney, Andes, & Blackwell, 2007). On the other hand, nurses as well as physiotherapists have more physically demanding work. In addition, physiotherapists are equipped with skills that let them spend their leisure time actively and they also have the need for movement, formed during their studies. Regular physical activity is declared by more than 50% of the respondents, 54% of students and 45% of professionals, including approximately 40% of physicians. The findings are similar to those obtained by Puciato, Rozpara, Mynarski, Łoś and Krolikowska (2013) for this professional group in Poland. Hence, it is hard to avoid the conclusion that, even though having appropriate health-related knowledge and beliefs about the crucial role of physical activity, the examined occupational groups (particularly physicians and nurses) don't implement them in their own personal lives (more than 50% of them). Conversely, American and Canadian physicians are more likely to be physically active than the general population (Frank et al., 2003, Frank & Segura, 2009).

Based on the analysis of the subjective and social determinants of physical activity among the respondents, it appears that the most important ones are as follows: high physical activity self-efficacy, low Chance Health Locus of Control, good Self-rated Health, BMI within a normal range and belonging to one of the studied socio-economic groups: physiotherapists or physiotherapy students. Taking into account that above mentioned determinants appear in the literature, the results are rather unsurprising. Exercise self-efficacy is revealed as the strongest predictor of continued exercise behaviour (Armitage & Conner, 2001). Self-rated Health is also a good predictor of physical activity, especially leisure time (Galána, Meseguer, Herruzo, & Rodriguez-Artalejo, 2010). Results in the studies investigating the relationships between the physical activity and health locus of control were similar, but not necessarily always the same. High Chance Health Locus of Control and high Powerful Others Health Locus of Control contribute to low physical activity while high Internal Health Locus of Control to high physical activity (Grotz, Hapke, Lampert, & Baumeister, 2011; Helmer, Krämer, & Mikolajczyk, 2012; Steptoe & Wardle, 2001).

From the perspective of a potential promotion programme directed to those socio-economic groups, the use of the skills and social competence training can be recommended, particularly focused on the belief in the possibility of dealing with potential obstacles in the organisation and implementation of physical activity necessary for various health benefits. Interestingly, a strong belief that our health does not depend on external factors such as chance or fate, strengthens the ability to cope with adversity and personal weakness in the moment of taking a challenge of increasing physical activity. The relationship between high Internal Health Locus of Control and physical activity is similar. These are not constructs which can be easily controlled or modified in adults. However, just facing the role of the mentioned psychological dispositions in personal decisions regarding health may be a valuable learning experience for the potential recipients of the programme, i.e. in this case, the future or present medical staff. Taking into account the predictive value associated with physical activity, the determination of Health Locus of Control should be also a part of assessment of the programme participants. The programmes dedicated to the increase of physical activity should be addressed in particular to such professional groups as physicians, nurses and medical students.

5.2 Nutrition

The nutrition behaviours of the respondents were analysed in two ways: taking 12 elements of proper diet into account (NI12) and taking 3 important diet elements, namely the consumption of vegetables, fruits and complex carbohydrates, into account (NI3). As it has been revealed, almost 60% of men and 65% of women in Poland consume fruits and vegetables on a daily basis – these results are close to the average for the population in Europe, whereas slightly more than 70% of the Polish population with higher education implements these recommendations (OECD, 2012). However, the research conducted by the Polish Public Opinion Research Center on a representative sample shows that the percentages are in fact much lower. In 2010 there was about 37% of those eating vegetables and 38% of those eating fruits every day (Dietary Behaviours and Eating Habits of Poles, 2010). In the group of present and future medical personnel, vegetables and fruits are consumed by 45% and 40%, respectively. The consumption of vegetables and fruits, as well as general eating habits, improve with the age of the respondents which is the opposite of what happens in relation to physical activity. College is a salient transition period for health behaviour change in young adults (Harris, Gordon-Larson, Chantala, & Udry, 2006). On the other hand, eating habits of students both in the US and in Europe get worse (Chourdakis et al., 2011; Deliens, Clarys, Van Hecke, De Bourdeaudhuij, & Deforche, 2013; Lloyd-Richardson, Lucero, DiBello, Jacobson, & Wing, 2008). This may partially be explained by the fact that students leave home, begin a more independent life away from their parents, experience more freedom in deciding about their own lifestyles, and hence, "get a taste of student life" (Deliens, Clarys, De Bourdeaudhuij, & Deforche, 2014). Medical students are expected to have better eating habits than non-medical students (Kagan & Squires, 1984). However, the research shows that the results may be quite opposite to what is expected (Sakamaki, Toyama, Amamoto, Liu, & Shinfuku, 2005).

The highest percentage of those consuming fruit and vegetables on a daily basis can be found among physicians while the average percentage is found among physiotherapists and the lowest percentage among nurses. The results obtained for physicians are definitely worse than those in the research by Gacek (2011), though she analysed mainly interns who are known as the best role models in terms of lifestyle. It is difficult to say whether current medical and physiotherapy students will eat better in the future. Having a more stable life as well as being economically established and being of a higher socio-economic status after commencing work, all contribute to healthier eating habits (Dijkstra, Neter, Brouwer, Huisman, & Visser, 2014; Giskes et al., 2006; Malon et al., 2010). However, based on the analysis of variability in health habits in the past 15 years among students of the University School of Physical Education in Poznań we can observe a slight downward trend which means a decrease in the number of people with a particularly beneficial lifestyle and an increase in the number with a moderately beneficial lifestyle. The percentages of students with visibly negative patterns are rather stable (Laudańska-Krzemińska, unpublished). At the same time, Polish students have worse health indicators than students in Western Europe (Steptoea & Wardle, 2001). As a result, it is difficult to draw any encouraging conclusions.

The highest percentage of those who adopt beneficial dietary patterns can be observed among the surveyed physicians and as regards the three main diet elements (NI3) also among physiotherapists. Is it enough to stand out in comparison to the population of working Poles? Depending on the research used as a point of reference, the comparison is very unfavourable (ODCE, 2012) for the surveyed personnel or moderately unfavourable (Dietary Behaviours and Eating

Habits of Poles, 2010). Irrespective of the point of reference, the adopted patterns of health behaviours can hardly be considered exemplary for patients or clients. US women physicians' diets were also worse than those of other women of high socio-economic status (Frank, Brogan, Mokdad, Simoes, Kahn, & Greenberg, 1998).

During the search for subjective and social determinants of eating habits in the group of medical personnel participating in the study, the following were shown to be the most significant ones: high nutrition self-efficacy, low Powerful Others Health Locus of Control, high Self-rated Health, BMI within normal limits, and belonging to one of the surveyed professional groups (nurses, physiotherapists, physicians). Just like in the case of physical activity, the results obtained confirm the factors indicated in the literature to be related to dietary habits of adults. Self-efficacy determines the initiation, maintenance and cessation of strategies or behaviours, thus being a good predictor of eating behaviour (Conn, 1997, Strecher, DeVellis, Becker, & Rosenstock, 1986). A study that focused on promotion of self-regulatory skills in severely obese adults found that as these skills increased, so did perceived self-efficacy in relation to controlled eating, which in turn was associated with BMI change (Annesi & Gorjala, 2010). Shaikh and colleques (2008) found strong evidence for self-efficacy, social support and knowledge as predictors of adult consumption of vegetables and fruits. Evidence from the literature on cognitive self-regulation suggests that there may be potential for people to learn to self-regulate better, both through training and controlled exposure techniques in order to support effective weight control, both in clinical and community settings (Johnson, Pratt, & Wardle, 2012). Higher Powerful Others Locus of Control and higher Chance Health Locus of Control are associated with not paying attention to health nutrition among German students (Helmer et al., 2012), but it was also demonstrated that high Internal Health Locus of Control was associated with better diet (Bennett, Moore, Smith, Murphy, & Smith, 1994). Persons with better eating habits, especially those who are not overweight or obese, tend to rate their health better (Molarius et al., 2006).

From the perspective of the promotion programme, a main focus should be on social competencies necessary to deal with obstacles to the implementation of beneficial eating habits. Interestingly, the respondents who reluctantly gave control over their health to medical service specialists (or who did not perceive such specialists as totally responsible for their health conditions), adopted better dietary habits, though this applies mainly to physicians and physiotherapists and rarely nurses. Therefore, the determination of health locus of control seems to be very well founded. A special promotional support is required by students in the fields subject to analysis. American trends show that even if indicators and effects of bad eating habits are observed slightly less often compared to the general population they are still only at a slightly lower level, which poses a big challenge from the perspective of health of health care workers (McNerney et al., 2007).

5.3 Smoking

Cigarette smoking is one of the most harmful habits. In Poland, intensive efforts to reduce its volume and toxicity were undertaken through invoking the relevant legislation and organising promotional campaigns. Over the past decade the number of smokers decreased by almost 14% (OECD, 2012). According to the OECD data, in 2010 approximately 24% of Poland's population smoke cigarettes (18% of women and 31% men). The study results of NATPOL 2011 are slightly higher - they show that 27% of residents smoke (23% of women and 31% men). Introducing a smoking ban in public places in 2010 also improved the situation. About 11% of people quit smoking alone or know people who quit smoking under the impact of the new legislation in this area (Postawy wobec palenia papierosów, 2012). However, despite some fluctuation (e.g. a decreasing percentage of men, but at the same time an increasing percentage of women), over the last few years roughly 30% of residents smoke.

Among the current and future medical staff respondents in this study, the observed trend is toward an increasing proportion of professionals who smoke, especially nurses. Similarly, negative results in this occupational group were obtained in studies run by Gańczak, Szych and Karakiewicz (2012) and Zysnarska, Bernad and Kara (2007) although the respondents in those studies grew up in conditions of greater social acceptance of smoking.

The proportion of daily smokers in the early 1990s was 51% among men and 25% among women (Stan zagrożenia, 2009). For young people at the time statistics were as follows: 50% of men and 30% of women. In the early 1980s the physician community stood out particularly negatively. Percentage values of smokers regarding gender among the group were, male physicians (43%) and female physicians (36%) – it was partially explained by poor knowledge about the negative health effects of smoking at that time. This situation began to improve in this professional group and in 2000 the percentage of smokers among physicians, in both sexes were: male physicians – 25% and female physicians – 15% (Stan zagrożenia, 2009). In the present study, as in Gańczak et al. (2012), there are 18% of smokers among physicians. Thus, we can expect favourable trends in cigarette smoking among current medical students. The increased rate of smoking in professionals probably results from their experiences in early youth and may not be prognostic for current medical students, the group with the percentage of smokers reaching approximately 14%. Comparing this study's results to the statistics about 5 years ago, a slight overall decline in smoking medical students (Siemińska et al., 2006) can be observed which is significantly lower than in the general population of students (where the rate is near 30%) (Rasińska & Nowakowska, 2012; Łaszek, Nowacka, & Szatko, 2011). Irrespective of that fact, the current medical staff being responsible for the health of Poles, especially nurses and physiotherapists, they do not compare favourably when it comes to their attitude towards smoking – the percentage of smokers in this group is similar to or even higher than average within the population of Poland (OECD, 2012). Lower percentages of smokers are also observed among physicians and physiotherapists from the United States, Canada and some Western European countries (Bazargan, Makar, Bazargan-Hejazi, Ani, & Wolf, 2009; Bolinder, Himmelmann, & Johansson, 2002; DuMonthier, Haneline, & Smith 2009; Frank & Segura 2009; Frank et al., 1998; Smith & Leggat, 2007). However, American medical students smoke more frequently than physicians (Hull, DiLalla, & Dorsey, 2008).

When it comes to social and subjective determinants that lead to tobacco addiction, the most important among the respondents is smoking self-efficacy, which is observed in other studies (Van Zundert, Ferguson, Shiffman, Saul, & Rutger, 2010). In contrast, we observe a different kind of relationship between low Powerful Others Health Locus of Control (related to the medical authorities' responsibility for our health) and smoking to which such low Powerful Others Health Locus of Control contributes. Faith in the specialists' assurances and the desire to entrust health to them help to avoid a smoking habit, similar to having a strong belief in personal responsibility for health. In the Grotz et al. (2011) study of smokers, those scoring high on the Powerful Others scale had made more attempts to stop smoking and persons scoring high on the Internal Scale smoked more frequently. In the studies conducted by Helmer et al. (2012) higher ratings in the Chance Health Locus of Control dimension were associated with a higher likelihood of being a current smoker. These inconsistencies in findings are in line with previous studies, which also found either insignificant or inconsistent results and rather small effects, especially for the internal dimension (Norman, Bennett, Smith, & Murphy, 1998; Steptoe & Wardle, 2001a; Wardle & Steptoe, 2003). As a result, these skills should be reinforced in educational programmes targeted especially to the current professionals.

5.4 Alcohol Consumption

Excessive alcohol use is associated with the negative health consequences, both in terms of morbidity and mortality (Rehm et al., 2009, WHO Europe, 2012a). In Europe, we note the highest rates of alcohol consumption in the world. In some countries it increases while decreases in other ones, hence the European mean is quite stable. In Poland, over the last 20 years a significant decrease in alcohol consumption was recorded (OECD, 2012). Unfavourable alcohol consumption particularly relates to young people currently studying (Karam, Kyprosd, & Marianac, 2007). On the one hand, it is quite characteristic of this period of life (Arnett, 2005; White, McMorris, Catalano, Fleming, Haggerty, & Abbott, 2006), on the other hand, it is a behaviour which leads to addiction. Among the students in this study, 38% of medical students and 28% of physiotherapy students admitted to the unfavourable pattern of alcohol consumption. These values are similar to those obtained by Łaszek et al. (2011) and much lower than the results of Bielska, Kurpas, Marcinowicz, Owłasiuk, Litwiejko and Wojtal (2012) – as measured by other research tools. In studies conducted on chiropractic students in the United States, binge drinking was also identified as a problem (DuMonthie et al., 2009, Baldwin et al., 2008). Harmful effects of alcohol consumption significantly less frequently occur among health professionals, which does not mean that it is a marginal problem as it relates to 21% of physicians and physiotherapists and 9% of nurses. In Poland, the number of addicted physicians may amount to approximately 12,000 (Woronowicz, 2010). In a study conducted at the Medical University of Poznan, more than 17% of employees declared alcohol consumption (Ziemska & Marcinkowski, 2010), with the rate in physicians of 28% (Ziemska, 2012). This is a very delicate and controversial subject, possibly even taboo for the medical community in Poland. Hazardous drinking among physicians (especially men) is also noticeable in the USA and Western Europe and concerns approximately 10% – 30% of them (McAuliffe, Rohman, Breer, Wyshak, Santangelo, & Magnuson, 1991; Oreskovich et al, 2012; Rosta & Aasland, 2013; Sebo, Gallacchi, Goehring, & Beat, 2007).

Among the social and subjective determinants investigated in the study, the most important are: alcohol self-efficacy, high Internal Health Locus of Control, high Chance Health Locus of Control and low Powerful Others Health Locus of Control. Findings indicate consistently that lower self-efficacy for avoiding alcohol is predictive of greater consumption (Atwell, Abraham, & Duka, 2011; Gilles, Turk, & Fresco, 2006). In the literature also the impact of these subjective competencies on alcohol consumption is highlighted. However, the results of different studies are not always consistent. For example, as the current studies have shown, a high Chance Health Locus of Control reduces the chance of risky drinking while in the studies of various groups of young people an inverse relationship was observed Helmer et al., 2012; Steptoe & Wardle, 2001b). The results of the current study were probably influenced by the dominance of this type of control among nurses, characterised by the highest proportion of alcohol abstainers. Similarly, in the study by Grotz et al. (2011) persons scoring high on the Internal Health Locus of Control Scale were less frequent consumers of moderate to higher levels of alcohol. The results of the Powerful Others Health Locus of Control Scale are also inconsistent. In this study, high Powerful Others Health Locus of Control score are associated with higher chances of risky drinking whereas in the study conducted by Steptoe and Wardle (2001b) high values on this scale implied a decrease in those chances. Again, it brings us to a conclusion that medical staff do not behave in accordance with generally observed trends in terms of control of health and its relationships with the selected behaviours, particularly the risky ones. In designing educational activities it is important to be very careful to tailor them to individual needs.

Promotion programmes concerning the excessive alcohol consumption can have a preventive character, but in the case of alcoholism the relevant treatment and therapeutic procedures are used while education plays here a supporting function. The current study gives recommendations for prevention programmes. In particular, it highlights the need to include the training of social competence and determination of the health locus of control in such programmes since people who have a strong sense of control over their own health or high Chance Health Locus of Control such as fate, God or divine forces abuse alcohol significantly less (this is especially the case amongst nurses). Also people who believe that their health does not depend on health professionals are less likely to have a tendency to abuse alcohol, too. Special care should be taken of medical students.

5.5 Co-Existence & Clusters

The study focused in particular on the identification and better understanding of relationships within multiple risk behaviours. It is one of the currently postulated directions of research exploration that is to facilitate more effective educational activities (Prochaska, 2014). As it has been revealed, a single behaviour-related risk factor in individuals is currently rare; it is more common to have a set of risk factors. Therefore, we should look for a common denominator for them in order to provide comprehensive therapeutic and educational solutions. As noticed by Leech Rebecca, McNaughton and Timperio (2014), we can distinguish two approaches to the analysis of multiple risk behaviours: co-existence and clustering. Both of them have advantages and limitations and therefore, both were used in this study. The theoretical background for such a search in this paper includes, for example, the Theory of Triadic Influence.

One of the results of this study that is worth noting is the percentage of people who accumulate beneficial and adverse health behaviours (taking the four studied behaviours into consideration). Only one in ten students and close to one in seven professionals accumulates all four beneficial health behaviours. It means that these individuals fully comply with the health recommendations that they should be promoting among their patients (clients). The accumulation of three beneficial behaviours in cross-sectional studies, for example among Hungarians, was reported in less than 6% of the respondents and of two behaviours in 25% of them (Paulik, Boka, Kertesz, Balogh, & Nagymajtenyi, 2010). Similarly, in the Danish population a full accumulation of health beneficial behaviours in respect of smoking, dietary patterns and physical activity was reported in 3% of the respondents (De Vries, Kremers, Smeets, & Reubsaet, 2008). As a counterbalance, we may present the percentage of the respondents who accumulate three or four health risk behaviours (low nutrition status, current smoking, low physical activity, heavy or binge alcohol consumption). At it has been revealed, we can observe several professionals accumulating all the four risk behaviours (1%) whereas three risk behaviours are accumulated by 6% of students and 11% of professionals. When we look further, it becomes clear that one in four students and one in five professionals accumulate two health risk behaviours.

Research on clustering has suggested that only a small proportion of the populations studied meet all (or almost all) of the recommended guidelines for the behaviours assessed (De Vries et al., 2008; Fine et al., 2004; Ford, Ford, Will, Galuska, & Ballew, 2001; Pronk et al., 2004; Schuit et al., 2002). Obviously, this fact suggests that necessary directions for action need to be taken, e.g. health promotion programmes.

In the search for patterns of accumulations typical for future and present medical personnel participating in the study, a statistical procedure different from the previously mentioned approach was used, namely cluster analysis, on the basis of which four clusters were distinguished. Cluster 2 was particularly interesting since it grouped individuals with a relatively good diet and high physical activity, being moderate alcohol drinkers and current non-smokers. Unfortunately, this pattern is followed only by 27%, i.e. one in four respondents. Next, another 27% of the respondents follow the moderate pattern (moderate diet, non-smoking, not abusing alcohol but also physically inactive). It seems then that not much is needed for them to follow the assumed beneficial pattern and an intervention is required to encourage an increase in everyday physical activity (cluster 4). The other two clusters contain almost a half of the respondents and are characterised by a poor diet, varied physical activity as well current/ex-smoking (cluster 3) or heavy/binge drinking (cluster 1) status. The cluster consisting of those with heavy/binge drinking status is most typical of students whereas the one characterised by smoking is typical of professionals. It is difficult to find role models for patients or clients among the persons, amounting to 46% of the respondents, who follow such behaviour patterns.

An analysis was performed on both social and subjective determinants of the distinguished clusters. Persons allocated to **cluster 1** rate their own health as moderate, health is not ranked high in their hierarchy of values, they do not appreciate their role in their own health care, entrust it to health specialists and do not believe that their health depends on fate or chance; moreover, most frequently they are overweight or their body weight is in the lower limit of normal. The persons allocated to **cluster 2** rate their own health as good or very good, health is an important value in their lives, they have a high sense of control over their own health, and thus, they believe that health care personnel controls it to a small extent and their BMI is generally normal. The persons allocated to **cluster 3** rate their health as bad, do not appreciate the value of health in life, they are not distinguishable in terms of health locus of control and most often they are overweight. The persons allocated to **cluster 4** rate their health as moderate, appreciate health as an important value in their lives, do not feel in control of their own health, entrust such control to health care specialists and believe that health depends also on external factors such as fate, chance or God, most often they are underweight or have normal body weight.

The following can be considered as psycho-social factors associated with beneficial patterns of health behaviours: valuation of health as an important value in life, high internal health locus of control (whereas high external health locus of control plays an ambivalent role), good or very good self-rated health. Self-rated health proves to be a predicator of health behaviour patterns beneficial to health and it is suggested that this measure should be more often used in the assessment of population health (Bopp, Braun, Gutzwiller, & Faeh, 2012; Tsai, Ford, Li, Zhao, Pearson, & Balluz, 2010; Wu, Wang, Zhao, Ma, Wu, Yan, & He, 2013). Generally, Internal Health Locus of Control is positively associated with health-enhancing behaviours, such as proper diet or physical activity, whereas Powerful Others or Chance Health Locus of Control are associated with risk behaviours, such as smoking or drinking alcohol. In this study a group particularly diverging from this pattern includes nurses, who form a professional group specifically succumbing to external control within the scope of health, both with reference to authorities and fate or chance, which does not prevent, and may even strengthen some of their choices beneficial to health, especially within the scope of alcohol consumption.

It should be also emphasised that, as other studies reveal, self-efficacy so significantly associated with the individual studied behaviours are also associated with each other, for example, self-efficacy for refraining from smoking was associated with self-efficacy for physical activity as well as self-efficacy for nutrition-related behaviours and physical activity (Boudreaux, Wood, Mehan, Scarinci,Taylor, & Brantley 2003; King, Marcus, Pinto, Emmons, & Abrams, 1996; Kremers et al., 2004). This fact also argues for searching multidimensional strategies for changing health risk behaviours.

The paper proposes also a construct of Health Behaviour Profiles (HBP), based on the division of the respondents' activities related to their own health (health enhancing behaviours and health-compromising behaviours) as a starting point. Five HBPs were distinguished on that basis: *destructive, passive, ambivalent, average and beneficial*. In this study a focus was on the issue of taking up both beneficial and adverse activities. With reference to physical activity and nutrition the activity means any action enhancing health whereas the situation is different for smoking and alcohol consumption. Here, it is "avoidance" and abstinence that are essential for health. On that basis the study revealed about 40% of persons representing the *beneficial* profile and 20% of persons with *average* profile. The remaining respondents (about 40%) represent adverse profiles, namely *destructive, passive* and *ambivalent*, including as many as 13% representing the first one. It is another confirmation that almost half of present and future health care specialists adopt an adverse lifestyle. This diversification, especially in terms of the frequency of representation of adverse profiles, can be also observed among students and professionals, where worse patterns are significantly more often observed among professionals.

While analyzing social and subjective correlates of the distinguished profiles, it can be concluded that they are differentiated by most of the variables subject to analysis. Representatives of the *beneficial* profile are characterised by the following: health is a significant personal value and an important prerequisite for personal happiness, they have a high sense of Internal Health Locus of Control and a low sense of Chance Health Locus of Control, they highly value their health potential and usually have a normal body weight. Representatives of the *average* profile are characterised by the following: health is a value of moderate importance to them, they have a high sense of Internal Health Locus of Control and a low sense of Chance Health Locus of Control, they rate their health as good and they usually have a normal body weight. Representatives of the *passive* profile are similar to those representing the *average* profile in terms of health valuation but they have a low sense of Internal Health Locus of Control and a high sense of Chance Health Locus of Control and they are quite often underweight. Representatives of the ambivalent profile are characterised by the following: ambivalent valuation of health (significant as a personal value, rather unimportant as a prerequisite for happiness), low rating of their own health, a low sense of both Internal Health Locus of Control and Chance Health Locus of Control. Representatives of the destructive profile are characterised by the following: health is a value not very important to them, their self-rated health is low, they have a low sense of Internal Health Locus of Control and a high sense of Chance Health Locus of Control and quite often they are overweight. The presented characteristics may form a basis for more precise adjustment of the promotional programme to the needs of participants, depending on the represented health behaviour profile.

The application of clustering of lifestyle factors is important because it may provide indications for more effective, lifestyle-based health promotion strategies than the more traditional single behaviour approach. Obviously, in order to do so, in-depth information needs to be gathered regarding a series of health behaviours, potentially leading to longer assessment procedures. However, an advantage of the lifestyle approach lies in the fact that offering a target group the possibility of choosing which health behaviour to improve, constitutes an attractive feature for intervention designers (De Vries et al., 2008). Moreover, when motivational stages and cognitive factors are found to cluster across health behaviours, a positive change in intrapersonal determinants of one behaviour might also induce changes in the related construct for another, clustered, behaviour (King et al., 1996; Kremers et al., 2004). Thus, the principle of these "synergistic" effects forms a potentially effective ingredient of health promotion programmes (Kremers et al., 2006).

6 Conclusion

There is increasing recognition of the importance of medical staff health. Large-scale programmes targeting life style behaviour analyses among current and future medical professionals are still required, in particular in East Central Europe, e.g. in Poland. In the present study, the level of implementation and co-occurrence of health behaviours among current and future health professionals were analysed. Their subjective and social determinants were also highlighted. By way of summary, the research questions will be answered.

Q1. The level of health behaviours presented by a large number of the studied current and prospective medical personnel does not support health. As regards physical activity, the studied physicians, nurses and medical students present the average level for the Polish population, which means that less than half of them present a high level of physical activity. Nutrition habits are unhealthy for one in three students and one in four professionals. The percentages of current or ex-smokers are lower or similar to the data for the population of Poland. Binge or high alcohol consumption are characteristic of one in three students and one in five professionals.

Q2. Differences between the studied groups in the co-occurrence of both adverse and beneficial behaviours are observed. It transpires that nurses, as a group, show more frequent accumulation of unhealthy behaviours. The highest number of people accumulating all beneficial behaviours is identified among physicians and physiotherapists. A higher physical activity level is associated with more beneficial nutrition, particularly among professionals (physiotherapists, nurses, physicians). It is also connected with the no smoking status, in particular among professionals (physicians and nurses). A better nutritional behaviour is associated with a more healthy level of alcohol consumption, especially among professionals (physiotherapists, physicians, nurses). It is also related to the no smoking status, especially among professionals (physiotherapists, physicians, nurses). Four clusters of health behaviours are identified. One of them is more often presented by students, and another – by professionals. Each cluster is typical for one or two groups of respondents (medical or physiotherapy students, physicians, nurses and physiotherapists). There is a difference between the groups of students and medical staff. Five Health Behaviour Profiles are analysed (*destructive, passive, ambivalent, average, beneficial*), which vary among the groups of respondents. The *destructive* profile is the most common among nurses, and the *beneficial* profile is the most common among physiotherapy students.

Q3. All the studied groups differ with respect to all health behaviours. Physiotherapy students are the most physically active, physicians and physiotherapists have the best nutrition habits, the lowest percentages of smoking habits are characteristic of physiotherapy students, the lowest rates of binge and high alcohol consumption typifies nurses. The studied groups have been found to differ with respect to almost all subject and biological variables.

Q4. Models of determination for all the investigated health behaviours are identified. Health-related self-efficacy is the most important variable correlated with all investigated health behaviours. Other important correlates are: health locus of control, self-rated health, BMI status and membership in one of the studied groups. The subject, biological and social variables correlated with the identified health behaviour clusters are: health locus of control, self-rated health, BMI status and membership in one of the studied groups.

The subject, biological and social variables which correlate with Health Behaviour Profiles are: self-rated health, valuation of health, Internal and Chance Health Locus of Control and BMI. The studied groups differ in respect to Health Behaviour Profiles.

Q5. Health related self-efficacy plays a mediator role in the relationship between health valuation and health behaviour only with respect to smoking (medium effect). Health related self-efficacy plays a mediator role in the relationship between health locus of control and health behaviour with respect to physical activity (small effect), nutrition (small effect) and smoking (large effect).

Q6. Health locus of control plays a mediator role in the relationship between health valuation and health behaviour with respect to physical activity (small effect), nutrition (small effect) and smoking (small effect).

The importance of health behaviours in the general population has been recognized and it is expected that health professionals will support their patients in healthy lifestyle choices. The preventive activities and healthy choices should be important for physicians, nurses and physiotherapists, too. There is a need for intervention targeting preventive health care issues, such as proper nutrition, increasing physical activity and quitting smoking, which could positively affect the personal health of medical staff and, as a consequence – their patients. The educational and behavioural needs of the investigated current and prospective medical personnel depend on career stage and profession. As a result, there is a need for health promotional programs targeting carefully chosen medical staff groups, with an emphasis on their special health needs. The expectation that physicians or other medical professionals will heal themselves proves to be futile. This point of view is also connected with the more general reflection on the health care system in Poland. Poland needs changes in health and social policies directed at preventive medicine, seen as a solution to better individual and social health, than at reactive medicine.

Bibliography

Abramson, S., Stein, J., Schaufele, M., Frates, E., & Rogan, S. (2000). Personal exercise, habits and counseling practices of primary care physicians: a national survey. *Clinical Journal of Sport Medicine, 10,* 40-48.

Ajzen, I. (1991). The theory of planned behavior. *Organizational Behavior and Human Decision Processes, 50,* 179–211.

Ajzen, I. (2002). Perceived behavioral control, self-efficacy, locus of control, and the theory of planned behavior. *Journal of Applied Social Psychology, 32,* 665-683.

Aktywność fizyczna Polaków. (2013). Komunikat z badań. CBOS. BS/129/2013, Centrum Badania Opinii Społecznej, Warszawa

Allegrante, J.P., Peterson, J.C., Boutin-Foster, C., Ogedegbe, G., & Charlson, M.E. (2008). Multiple health-risk behavior in a chronic disease population: what behaviors do people choose to change? *Preventive Medicine, 46,* 247-251.

Amarowicz, R., & Pegg, R.B. (2008). Legumes as a source of natural antioxidants. *European Journal of Lipid Science and Technology, 110,* 865-878.

Anderson, P. & Baumberg, B. (2006). *Alcohol in Europe.* London: Institute of Alcohol Studies.

Annesi, J.J., & Gorjala, S. (2010). Relations of self-regulation and self-efficacy for exercise and eating and BMI change: a field investigation. *Biopsychosocial Medicine, 4,* 10.

Anokye, N.K., Trueman, P., Green, C., Pavey, T.G., & Taylor, R.S. (2012). Physical activity and health related quality of life. *BMC Public Health, 12,* 624.

Armitage, C.J., & Conner, M. (2001). Efficacy of the theory of planed behavior: a meta-analytic review. *British Journal of Social Psychology, 40,* 471-499.

Arnett, J.J. (2005). The developmental context of substance use in emerging adulthood. *Journal of Drug Issues, 35,* 235-254.

Atkinson, R., & Flint, J. (2001). Accessing hidden and hard-to-reach populations: snowball research strategies. *Social Research Update, 33.*

Attitudes of Europeans towards tobacco. (2012). Special Eurobarometer 385/Wave EB77.1 – TNS Opinion & Social

Atwell, K., Abraham, C., & Duka, T. (2011). A parsimonious, integrative model of key psychological correlates of UK university students' alcohol consumption. *Alcohol and Alcoholism, 46(3),* 253-260.

Babor, T.F., & Higgins-Biddle, J.C. (2001). Brief Intervention for hazardous and harmful drinking: a manual for use in primary care. World Health Organization.

Babor, T.F., Higgins-Biddle, J.C., Saunders, J.B., & Monteiro, M.G. (2001). Audit: the alcohol use disorders identification test guidelines for use in primary care. World Health Organization.

Baldwin, J.N., Davis-Hall, R.E., DeSimone, E.M., Scott, D.M., Agrawal, S., & Reardon, T.P. (2008). Survey of attitudes and behaviors toward alcohol and other drug use in allied health and physician assistant students. *Journal of Allied Health, 37,* 156-161.

Bandura, A. (1977). Self-efficacy: toward a unifying theory of behavioral change. *Psychology Review, 84,* 191-215.

Bandura, A. (1986). *Social foundations of thought and action: A social cognitive theory.* Prentice-Hall, Englewood Cliffs, NJ.

Bandura, A. (2001). Social cognitive theory: An agentive perspective. *Annual Review of Psychology, 52(1),* 1-26.

Baron, R.M., & Kenny, D.A. (1986). The moderator-mediator variable distinction in social psychological research: conceptual, strategic, and statistical considerations. *Journal of Personality and Social Psychology, 51,* 1173-1182.

Bazargan, M., Makar, M., Bazargan-Hejazi, S., Ani, C., & Wolf, K.E. (2009). Preventive, lifestyle, and personal health behaviors among physicians. *Academic Psychiatry, 33(4),* 289-295.

Bazzano, L.A., Thompson, A.M., Tees, M.T., Nguyen, C.H., & Winham, D.M. (2011). Non-soy legume consumption lowers cholesterol levels: a meta-analysis of randomized controlled trials. *Nutrition, Metabolism & Cardiovascular Diseases, 21(2),* 94-103.

Becker, M.H. (1974). *The health belief model and personal health behavior.* Thorofare, NJ: Slack.

Bennett, P., Moore, L., Smith, A., Murphy, S., & Smith, C. (1994). Health locus of control and value for health as predictors of dietary behavior. *Psychology & Health, 10(1),* 41-54.

Bielska, D., Kurpas, D., Marcinowicz, L., Owłasiuk, A., Litwiejko, A., & Wojtal, M. (2012). Evaluation of the risk of alcohol consumption and tobacco smoking among 6th year students of the Faculty of Medicine. *Przegląd Lekarski, 69,* 10.

Biernat, E., & Stupnicki, R. (2005). An overview of internationally applicable questionnaires designed for assessing physical activity. *Physical Education and Sport, 49,* 32-42.

Biondi-Zoccai, G.G., Abbate, A., Liuzzo, G., & Biasucci, L.M. (2003). Atherothrombosis, inflammation, and diabetes. *Journal of the American College of Cardiology, 41(7),* 1071-1077.

Blair, S.N., LaMonte, M.J., & Nichaman, M.Z. (2004). The evolution of physical activity recommendations: how much is enough? *The American Journal of Clinical Nutrition, 79,* 913-920.

Boden, J.M., & Fergusson, D.M. (2011). Alcohol and depression. *Addiction, 106,* 906-914.

Bolinder, G., Himmelmann, L., & Johansson, K. (2002). Swedish physicians smoke least in all the world. A new study of smoking habits and attitudes to tobacco. *Lakartidningen, 99(30-31),* 3111-3117.

Bopp, M., Braun, J., Gutzwiller, F., & Faeh, D. (2012). Health risk or resource? Gradual and independent association between self-rated health and mortality persists over 30 years. *PLoS ONE, 7(2).*

Boudreaux, E.D., Wood, K.B., Mehan, D., Scarinci I., Taylor, C.L., & Brantley, P.J. (2003). Congruence of readiness to change, self-efficacy, and decisional balance for physical activity and dietary fat reduction. *American Journal of Health Promotion, 17(5),* 329-336.

Breslow, J.L. (2006). N-3 fatty acids and cardiovascular disease. *The American Journal of Clinical Nutrition, 83,* 1477-1482.

Bronfenbrenner, M. (1986). Ecology of the family as a context for human development: research perspectives. *Developmental Psychology, 22,* 723-742.

Brunner, E.J., Mosdøl, A., Witte, D.R., Martikainen, P., Stafford, M., Shipley, M.J., & Marmot, M.G. (2008). Dietary patterns and 15-y risks of major coronary events, diabetes, and mortality. *American Journal of Clinical Nutrition, 87,* 1414-1421.

Cade, J.E., Burley, V.J., Greenwood, D.C., & UK Women's Cohort Study Steering Group (2007). Dietary fibre and risk of breast cancer in the UK Women's Cohort Study. *International Journal of Epidemiology, 36(2),* 431-438.

Capra, F. (1982). *The turning point: science, society, and the rising culture.* Simon and Schuster.

Caspersen, C.J., Powell, K.E., & Christensen, G.M. (1985). Physical activity, exercise, and physical fitness: definitions and distinctions for health-related research. *Public Health Reports, 100,* 126-131.

CDC. *Fact Sheets - Preventing Excessive Alcohol Use.* (n.d.). Retrieved from: http://www.cdc.gov/alcohol/fact-sheets/prevention.htm

Chanson-Rollé, A., Lappi, J., Meynier, A., Poutanen, K., Vinoy, S., & Braesco, V. (2014). Health benefits of wholegrain; a systematic review of the evidence to propose a daily intake recommendation. *The FASEB Journal, 28,* 1.

Chien-Ning, T., Bih-Shya, G., & Meei-Fang, L. (2011). The effectiveness of exercise on improving cognitive function in older people: a systematic review. *Journal of Nursing Research, 19(2),* 119-131.

Chmiel, J., Chołuj, K., Fijewski, A., & Mjcher, P. (2009). Analiza porównawcza zdolności motorycznych studentów I roku fizjoterapii i farmacji Uniwersytetu Medycznego w Lublinie oraz ich opinii dotyczących sprawności fizycznej w przyszłej pracy zawodowej. *Zdrowie Publiczne, 119(4),* 417-420.

Cho, E., Seddon, M., Rosner, B., Willett, C., & Hankinson, E. (2004). Prospective study of intake of fruits, vegetables, vitamins, and carotenoids and risk of age-related maculopathy. *Archive of Ophthalmology, 122,* 883-892.

Chourdakis, M., Tzellos, T., Pourzitaki, C., Toulis, K.A., Papazisis, G., & Kouvelas, D. (2011). Evaluation of dietary habits and assessment of cardiovascular disease risk factors among Greek university students. *Appetite, 57(2),* 377-383.

Chowdhury, R., Stevens, S., Gorman, D., Pan, A., Warnakula, S., Chowdhury, S., ... Franco, O.H. (2012). Association between fish consumption, long chain omega 3 fatty acids, and risk of cerebrovascular disease: systematic review and meta-analysis. *BMJ,* 345.

Cohen, J. (1988). *Statistical power analysis for the behavioral sciences,* 2nd ed., Hillsdale, NJ.

Conn, V.S. (1997). Older women. Social cognitive theory correlates of health behavior. *Women and Health, 26,* 71-85.

Corrao, G., Bagnardi, V., Zambon, A., & La Vecchia, C. (2004). A meta-analysis of alcohol consumption and the risk of 15 diseases. *Preventive Medicine, 38,* 613-619.

Cotter, K.A., & Lachman, M.E. (2010). No strain, no gain: psychosocial predictors of physical activity across the adult lifespan. *Journal of Physical Activity and Health, 7,* 584-594.

Council conclusions on nutrition and physical activity. Council of the European Union. (2014). *Official Journal of the European Union, 213*(1), Retrived from: http://eur-lex.europa.eu/legal-content/EN/TXT/PDF/?uri=CELEX:52014XG0708%2801%29&rid=14

Craig, C.L., Marshall, A.L., Sjöström, M., Bauman, A.E., Booth, M.L., Ainsworth, B.E., ... Oja, P. (2003). International physical activity questionnaire: 12-country reliability and validity. *Medicine & Science in Sports & Exercise, 35(8),* 1381-1395.

Dahm, C.C., Keogh, R.H., Spencer, E.A., Greenwood, D.C., Key, T.J., Fentiman, I.S., ... Rodwell Bingham, S.A. (2010). Dietary fiber and colorectal cancer risk: a nested case-control study using food diaries. *Journal of the National Cancer Institute, 102(9),* 614-626.

Dauchet, L., Amouyel, P., & Dallongeville, J. (2005). Fruit and vegetable consumption and risk of stroke: a meta-analysis of cohort studies. *Neurology, 65,* 1193-1197.

De Vries, H., Kremers, S., Smeets, T., & Reubsaet, A. (2008). Clustering of diet, physical activity and smoking and a general willingness to change. *Psychology and Health, 23(3),* 265-278.

Deliens, T., Clarys, P., De Bourdeaudhuij, I., & Deforche, B. (2014). Determinants of eating behaviour in university students: a qualitative study using focus group discussions. *BMC Public Health,* 14, 53.

Deliens, T., Clarys, P., Van Hecke, L., De Bourdeaudhuij, I., & Deforche, B. (2013). Changes in weight and body composition during the first semester at university. A prospective explanatory study. *Appetite, 65C,* 111-116.

Dietary Guidelines for Americans 2010. (2010) U.S. Department of Agriculture. U.S. Department of Health and Human Services. Retrieved from: http://www.health.gov/dietaryguidelines/dga2010/DietaryGuidelines2010.pdf

Dijkstra, S.C., Neter, J.E., Brouwer, I.A., Huisman, M., & Visser, M. (2014). Adherence to dietary guidelines for fruit, vegetables and fish among older Dutch adults; the role of education, income and job prestige. *The Journal of Nutrition, Health & Aging, 18(2),* 115-121.

Dinas, P. C., Koutedakis, Y., & Flouris, A.D. (2011). Effects of exercise and physical activity on depression. *Irish Journal of Medical Science, 180(2),* 319-325.

Dishman, R.K., Berthoud, H.R., Booth, F.W., Cotman, C.W., Edgerton, V.R., Fleshner, M.R., ... Zigmond, M.J. (2006). *Neurobiology of exercise. Obesity (Silver Spring), 14,* 345-356.

Dowda, M., Ainsworth, B.E., Addy, C.L., Saunders, R., & Riner, W. (2003). Correlates of physical activity among U.S. young adults, 18 to 30 years of age, from NHANES III. *Annals of Behavioral Medicine, 26,* 15-23.

Dube, A.R. & Stanton, C.A. (2010). The social context of dietary behaviors: the role of social relationships and support on dietary fat and fiber intake In F. De Meester et al. (Eds.), *Modern Dietary Fat Intakes in Disease Promotion, Nutrition and Health* (pp. 31-42). Springer Science+Business Media, DOI 10.1007/978-1-60327-571-2_2

Dufour, M. (1999). What is moderate drinking? Defining "drinks" and drinking levels. *Alcohol Research and Health, 23(1),* 5-14.

DuMonthier, W.N., Haneline, M.T., & Smith, M. (2009). Survey of health attitudes and behaviors of a chiropractic college population. *Journal of Manipulative and Physiological Therapeutics, 32,* 477-484.

Durstine, J.L., Grandjean, P.W., Cox, C.A., & Thompson, P.D. (2002).Lipids, lipoproteins, and exercise. *Journal of Cardiopulmonary Rehabilitation and Prevention, 22,* 385-398.

Dusseldorp, L., Velderman, M.K., Paulussen, T., Junger, M., van Nieuwenhuijzen, M., & Reijneveld, S.A. (2014). Targets for primary prevention: cultural, social and intrapersonal factors associated with co-occurring health-related behaviours. *Psychology & Health, 29(5),* 598-611.

Edington, D. W. (2001). Emerging research: a view from one research center. American Journal of Health Promotion, 15, 341–349.

Edington, D.W., Yen, L.T., & Witting, P. (1997). The financial impact of the changes in personal health practices. *Journal of Occupational and Environmental Medicine, 39,* 1037-1046.

Elwood, P.C., Pickering, J.E., Givens, D.I., & Gallacher, J.E. (2010). The consumption of milk and dairy foods and the incidence of vascular disease and diabetes: an overview of the evidence. *Lipids, 45,* 925-939.

Emmons, K.M., Marcus, B.H., Linnan, L., Rossi, J.S., & Abrams, D.B. (1994). Mechanisms in multiple risk factor interventions: smoking, physical activity, and dietary fat intake among manufacturing workers. *Preventive Medicine, 23,* 481-489.

EU Physical Activity Guidelines Recommended Policy Actions in Support of Health-Enhancing Physical Activity. (2008), WHO.

Fine, L., Philogene, G., Gramling, R., Coups, E., & Sinha, S. (2004). Prevalence of multiple chronic disease risk factors. 2001 National Health Interview Survey. *American Journal of Preventive Medicine, 27,* 18–24.

Flay, B.R., & Petraitis, J. (1994). The theory of triadic influence: A new theory of health behavior with implications for preventive interventions. *Advances in Medical Sociology, 4,* 19-44.

Flay, B.R., Snyder, F., & Petraitis, J. (2009). The theory of triadic influence. In: R.J. DiClemente, M.C. Kegler, R.A. Crosby (Eds.): *Emerging Theories in Health Promotion Practice and Research.* (pp 451-510). San Francisco: Jossey-Bass.

Ford, E.S., Ford, M.A., Will, J.C., Galuska, D.A., & Ballew, C. (2001). Achieving a healthy lifestyle among United States adults: A long way to go. *Ethnicity and disease, 11,* 224-231.

Frank, E., & Segura, C. (2009). Health practices of Canadian physicians. *Canadian Family Physician, 55(8),* 810-811.

Frank, E., Bhat, S.K., & Elon, L. (2003). Exercise counseling and personal exercise habits of US women physicians. *Journal of the American Medical Women's Association, 58,* 178-184.

Frank, E., Brogan, D.J., Mokdad, A.H., Simoes, E.J., Kahn, H.S., & Greenberg, R.S. (1998). Health-related behaviors of women physicians vs other women in the United States. *Archives of Internal Medicine, 158(4),* 342-348.

Freedman, N.D., Cross, A.J., McGlynn, K.A., Abnet, C.C., Park, Y., Hollenbeck, A.R., ... Sinha, R. (2010). Association of meat and fat intake with liver disease and hepatocellular carcinoma in the NIH-AARP cohort. *Journal of the National Cancer Institute, 102(17),* 1354-1365.

Fumeron, F., Lamri, A., Khalil, C.A., Jaziri, R., Porchay-Baldérelli, I., Lantieri, O., ... Marre, M. (2011). Dairy consumption and the incidence of hyperglycemia and the metabolic syndrome. Results from a French prospective study, Data from the Epidemiological Study on the Insulin Resistance Syndrome (DESIR). *Diabetes Care, 34,* 813-817.

Gacek, M. (2011). Eating behaviors and physical activity in a group of physicians. *Problemy Higieny i Epidemiologii, 92(2),* 254-259.

Galán, I., Meseguer, C.M., Herruzo, R., & Rodríguez-Artalejo, F. (2010). Self-rated health according to amount, intensity and duration of leisure time physical activity. *Preventive Medicine, 51(5),* 378-383.

Gańczak, M., Szych, Z., Karakiewicz, B. (2012). Tobacco smoking among doctors and nurses from surgical wards. *Hygeia Public Health, 47(1),* 72-76.

Garber, C.E., Blissmer, B., Deschenes, M.R., Franklin, B.A., Lamonte, M.J., Lee, I., ... Swain, D.P. (2011). Quantity and quality of exercise for developing and maintaining cardiorespiratory, musculoskeletal, and neuromotor fitness in apparently healthy adults: guidance for prescribing exercise. *Medicine and Science in Sports and Exercise, 43(7),* 1334-1359.

Gidding, S.S., Lichtenstein, A.H., Faith, M.S., Karpyn, A., Mennella, J.A., Popkin, B., ... Whitsel, L. (2009). Implementing American Heart Association pediatric and adult nutrition guidelines: a scientific statement from the American Heart Association Nutrition Committee of the Council on Nutrition, Physical Activity and Metabolism, Council on Cardiovascular Disease in the Young, Council on Arteriosclerosis, Thrombosis and Vascular Biology, Council on Cardiovascular Nursing, Council on Epidemiology and Prevention, and Council for High Blood Pressure Research. *Circulation, 119,* 1161-1175.

Gil, A., Ortega, R.M., & Maldonado J. (2011). Wholegrain cereals and bread: a duet of the Mediterranean diet for the prevention of chronic diseases. *Public Health Nutrition, 14(12A),* 2316-2322.

Gilles, D.M., Turk, C.L., & Fresco, D.M. (2006). Social anxiety, alcohol expectancies, and self-efficacy as predictors of heavy drinking in college students. *Addictive Behaviors, 31,* 388–98.

Giskes, K., Turrell, G., van Lenthe, F.J., Brug, J., & Mackenbach, J.P. (2006). A multilevel study of socio-economic inequalities in food choice behaviour and dietary intake among the Dutch population: the GLoBE study. *Public Health Nutrition, 9(1),* 75-83.

Glanz, K., Rimer, B.K., & Viswanath, K. (2008). *The scope of health behavior and health education in health behavior and health education theory, research, and practice 4th Edition.* Jossey-Bass A Wiley Imprint.

Global recommendations on physical activity for health. (2010). Geneva: World Health Organization, Retrived from: http://whqlibdoc.who.int/publications/2010/9789241599979_eng.pdf

Global status report on alcohol and health. (2014). Geneva: World Health Organization, Retrived from: http://www.who.int/substance_abuse/publications/global_alcohol_report/en/

Gniazdowski, A., Kopias, J., Korzeniowska, E., Nosko, J., Piwowarska-Pościk, L., & Puchalski, K. (1990). *Zachowania zdrowotne. Zagadnienie teoretyczne, próba charakterystyki zachowań zdrowotnych społeczeństwa polskiego.* Instytut Medycyny Pracy im. prof. J. Nofera, Łódź

Gochman, D.S. (Ed.). (1998). *Health Behavior Emerging Research Perspectives.* Springer Science & Business Media.

Golden Charter of Proper Nutrition (1997). *Czynniki ryzyka, Pismo Polskiego Towarzystwa Badań nad Miażdżycą, 3-4*

Gonçalves, A.K., Dantas Florêncio, G.L., de Atayde Silva, M.J.M., Cobucci, R.N., Giraldo, P.C., & Cote, N.M. (2014). Effects of physical activity on breast cancer prevention: a systematic review. *Journal of Physical Activity and Health, 11,* 445-454.

Graham, I., Atar, D., Borch-Johnsen, K., Boysen, G., Burell, G., Cifkova, R., ... Zampelas, A. (2007). European guidelines on cardiovascular disease prevention in clinical practice: executive summary: Fourth Joint Task Force of the European Society of Cardiology and Other Societies on

Cardiovascular Disease Prevention in Clinical Practice (Constituted by representatives of nine societies and by invited experts). *European Journal of Cardiovascular Prevention & Rehabilitation, 28,* 2375-2414.

Green paper on promoting healthy diets and physical activity: a European dimension for the prevention of overweight, obesity and chronic diseases, Commission of The European Communities. (2005). Brussels: Commission of The European Communities Retrieved from: http://eur-lex.europa.eu/legal-content/EN/TXT/PDF/?uri=CELEX:52005DC0637&from=EN

Grotz, M., Hapke, U., Lampert, T., & Baumeister, H. (2011). Health locus of control and health behaviour: results from a nationally representative survey. *Psychology, Health & Medicine, 16(2),* 129-140.

Gullone, E., & Moore, S. (2000). Adolescent risk-taking and the five-factor model of personality. *Journal of Adolescence, 23,* 393–407.

Hardeman, W., Johnston, M., Johnston, D., Bonetti, D., Wareham, N., & Kinmonth, A.L. (2002). Application of the Theory of Planned Behaviour in Behaviour Change Interventions: A Systematic Review. *Psychology & Health, 17(2),* 123-158.

Harris, K.M., Gordon-Larson, P., Chantala, K., & Udry, J.R. (2006). Longitudinal trends in race/ethnic disparities in leading health indicators from adolescence to young adulthood. *Archives of Pediatric Adolescent Medicine, 160,* 74-81.

Hash, R.B., Munna, R.K., Vogel R.L., & Bason J.J. (2003). Does physician weight affect perception of health advice? *Preventive Medicine, 36,* 41-44.

Hauner, H., Bechthold, A., Boeing, H., Brönstrup, A., Buyken, A., Leschik-Bonnet, E., ... Wolfram, G. (2012). Evidence-based guideline of the German Nutrition Society: carbohydrate intake and prevention of nutrition-related diseases. *Annals of Nutrition and Metabolism, 60(1),* 1-58.

Hawk, C., Long, C.R., Perillo, M., & Boulanger, K.T. (2004). A survey of US chiropractors on clinical preventive services. *Journal of Manipulative and Physiological Therapeutics, 27(5),* 287-298.

Hayes, A.F. (2009). Beyond Baron and Kenny: Statistical mediation analysis in the new millennium. *Communication Monographs, 76,* 408-420.

Hayes, A.F. (2013). *Introduction to mediation, moderation, and conditional process analysis.* New York: The Guilford Press

Hayes, A.F., & Preacher, K.J. (2010). Quantifying and testing indirect effects in simple Mediation models when the constituent paths are nonlinear. *Multivariate Behavioral Research, 45,* 627-660.

He, J., Nowson, A., Lucas, M., & MacGregor, A. (2007). Increased consumption of fruit and vegetables is related to a reduced risk of coronary heart disease: meta-analysis of cohort studies. *Journal of Human Hypertension, 21,* 717-728.

Health 2020. Leadership for health and well-being in 21st century Europe. (2012). World Health Organization, Retrived from: http://www.who.int/workforcealliance/knowledge/resources/Health2020_short.pdf?ua=1

Healthy Eating Pyramid. (2009). Instytut Zywnosci i Zywienia. Retrieved from: http://www.izz.waw.pl/pl/zasady-prawidowego-ywienia#c

Healthy People 2010. Final Review (2012). M.D. Hyattsville (Ed), National Center for Health Statistics. Retrieved from: http://www.cdc.gov/nchs/healthy_people/hp2010/hp2010_final_review.htm

Healthy People. The Surgeon General's Report On Health Promotion And Disease Prevention. (1979). U.S. Department Of Health, Education, And Welfare, Washington

Heidemann, C., Schulze, M.B., Franco, O.H., van Dam, R.M., Mantzoros, C.S., & Hu, F.B. (2008). Dietary patterns and risk of mortality from cardiovascular disease, cancer, and all causes in a prospective cohort of women. *Circulation, 118,* 230–237

Helmer, S.M., Krämer, A., & Mikolajczyk, R.T. (2012). Health-related locus of control and health behaviour among university students in North Rhine Westphalia, Germany. *BMC Research Notes, 5,* 703.

Heszen-Niejodek, I. (1997). Psychologiczne modele teoretyczne leżące u podstaw promocji zdrowia. In: Z., Ratajczak, I. & Heszen- Niejadek (Eds.). *Promocja zdrowia. Psychologiczne podstawy wdrożeń*. (pp.11-33), Wydawnictwo Uniwersytetu Śląskiego, Katowice.

Hetherington, M.M., Anderson, A.S., Norton, G.N., & Newson, L. (2006). Situational effects on meal intake: A comparison of eating alone and eating with others. *Physiology & Behavior, 88,* 498-505.

Hooper, L. (2007). Primary Prevention of CVD: diet and weight loss. *Clinical Evidence (online), 1.*

Hosseinpour-Niazi, S., Mirmiran, P., Sohrab, G., Hosseini-Esfahani, F., & Azizi, F. (2011). Inverse association between fruit, legume, and cereal fiber and the risk of metabolic syndrome: Tehran lipid and glucose study. *Diabetes Research and Clinical Practice, 94,* 276-283.

Housman, J., & Dorman, S. (2005). The alameda county study: a systematic, chronological review. *American Journal of Health Education, 36(5),* 302-308.

Howe, M., Leidel, A., Sangeetha M.K., Weber, A., Rubenfire, M., & Jackson E.A. (2010). Patient-related diet and exercise counseling: do providers' own lifestyle habits matter? *Preventive Cardiology, 13,* 180-185.

Hu, F.B. (2002). Dietary pattern analysis: a new direction in nutritional epidemiology. *Current Opinion in Lipidology, 13,* 3-9.

Hu, F.B., Stampfer, M.J., Manson, J.E., Rimm, E., Colditz, G.A., Rosner, B.A., ... Willett, W.C. (1997). Dietary fat intake and the risk of coronary heart disease in women. *The New England Journal of Medicine, 337,* 1491-1499.

Hull, S.K., DiLalla, L.F., & Dorsey, J.K. (2008). Prevalence of health-related behaviors among physicians and medical trainees. *Academic Psychiatry, 32(1),* 31-38.

Indulski J., & Leowski J. (1971), *Podstawy medycyny społecznej*, Warszawa: PZWL.

IPAQ (n.d.) International Physical Activity Questionaire. Retrieved from: http://www.ipaq.ki.se/downloads.htm

Irwin, C.E., & Millstein, S.G. (1986). Biopsychosocial correlates of risk-taking behaviors during adolescence: can the physician intervene? *Journal of Adolescence Health Care, 7,* 82-96.

Irwin, C.E., Igra, V., Eyre, S., & Millstein, S. (1997). Risk-taking behavior in adolescents: the paradigm. *Annals New York Academy Sciences, 28,* 1-35.

Isharwal, S., Misra, A., Wasir, J.S., & Nigam, P. (2009). Diet and insulin resistance: a review and Asian Indian perspective. *Indian Journal of Medical Research, 129,* 485-499.

Jessor, R. (1991). Risk behavior in adolescence: A psychosocial framework for understanding and action. *Journal of Adolescent health, 2,* 597–605.

Johnson, F., Pratt, M., & Wardle, J. (2012). Dietary restraint and self-regulation in eating behavior. *International Journal of Obesity, 36,* 665-674.

Juczyński, Z. (2001). *Narzędzia pomiaru w promocji i psychologii zdrowia*. Pracowania Testów Psychologicznych Wyd. PTP, Warszawa.

Kagan, D.M., & Squires, R.L. (1984). Compulsive eating, dieting, stress and hostility among college students. *Journal of College Student Personnel, 25(3),* 213-220.

Kaluza, J., Wolk, A., & Larsson, S.C. (2012). Red meat consumption and risk of stroke. A meta-analysis of prospective studies. *Stroke, 43,* 2556-2560.

Kant, A.K. (2004). Dietary patterns and health outcomes. *Journal of the American Dietetic Association, 104,* 615-635.

Kappeler, R., Eichholzer, M., & Rohrmann, S. (2013). Meat consumption and diet quality and mortality in NHANES III. *European Journal of Clinical Nutrition 67,* 598-606.

Karam, E., Kypri, K., & Salamoun, M. (2007). Alcohol use among college students: an international perspective. *Current Opinion in Psychiatry, 20(3),* 213-221.

Kickbusch, I., Pelikan, J.M., Apfel, F., & Tsouros, A.D. (Eds.) (2013) *Health literacy. The solid facts.* WHO Regional Office for Europe, Retrieved from: http://www.euro.who.int/__data/assets/pdf_file/0008/190655/e96854.pdf

King, B., & Minium, E. (2009). *Statystyka dla psychologów i pedagogów*. Warszawa: Wydawnictwo Naukowe PWN.

King, T., Marcus, B., Pinto, B., Emmons, K., & Abrams, D. (1996). Cognitive-behavioral mediators of changing multiple behaviors: smoking and a sedentary lifestyle. *Preventive Medicine, 25,* 684-691.

Kolbe, L.J. (1998). The Application of Health Behavior Research In D.S. Gohman (Ed.) *Health Behavior.* Springer US.

Kolonel, L.N., Hankin, J.H., Whittemore, A.S., Wu, A.H., Gallagher, R.P., Wilkens, L.R., … Paffenbarger, R.S. Jr. (2000). Vegetables, fruits, legumes and prostate cancer: a multiethnic case-control study. *Cancer Epidemiology, Biomarkers & Prevention, 9,* 795-804.

Korzeniowska, E. (1997). *Zachowania i świadomość zdrowotna w sferze pracy*. Instytut Medycyny Pracy, Łódź.

Kratz, M., Baars, T., & Guyenet, S. (2013). The relationship between high-fat dairy consumption and obesity, cardiovascular, and metabolic disease. *European Journal of Nutrition 52(1),* 1-24.

Kremers, S., De Bruijn, G., Schaalma, H., & Brug, J. (2004). Clustering of energy balance-related behaviours and their intrapersonal determinants. *Psychology and Health, 19,* 595–606.

Kremers, S., De Bruijn, G., Visscher, T., Van Mechelen, W., De Vries, N., & Brug, J. (2006). Environmental influences on energy balance-related behaviors: a dual-process view. *International Journal of Behavioral Nutrition and Physical Activity, 15,* 3-9.

Kris-Etherton, P.M., & Innis, S. (2007). Position of the American Dietetic Association and Dietitians of Canada: dietary fatty acids. *Journal of the American Dietetic Association 107(9),* 1599-1611.

Kris-Etherton, P.M., Harris, W.S., & Appel, L.J. (2002). Fish consumption, fish oil, omega-3 fatty acids, and cardiovascular disease. *Circulation, 106,* 2747-2757.

Lalonde, M. (1974). *A new perspective on the health of Canadians. A working document.* Ottawa: Government of Canada.

Langsetmo, L., Hitchcock, C.L., Kingwell, E.J., Davison, K.S., Berger, C., Forsmo, S., … Prior, J.C. (2012). Physical activity, body mass index and bone mineral density-associations in a prospective population-based cohort of women and men: The Canadian Multicentre Osteoporosis Study (CaMos). *Bone, 50(1),* 401-408.

Larsson, S.C., & Orsini, N. (2011). Fish consumption and the risk of stroke: a dose–response meta-analysis. *Stroke, 42,* 3621-3623.

Larsson, S.C., Virtamo, J., & Wolk, A. (2011a). Red meat consumption and risk of stroke in Swedish men. *The American Journal of Clinical Nutrition, 94,* 417-421.

Larsson, S.C., Virtamo, J., & Wolk, A. (2011b). Red meat consumption and risk of stroke in Swedish women. *Stroke, 42,* 324-329.

Łaszek, M., Nowacka, E., & Szatko, F. (2011). Negative behavior patterns of students. Part I. Consumption of alcohol and use of psychoactive substances. *Problemy Higieny i Epidemiologii, 92(1),* 114-119.

Lee, I., Shiroma, E.J., Lobelo, F., Puska, P., Blair, S.N., & Katzmarzyk, P.T. (2012). Effect of physical inactivity on major non-communicable diseases worldwide: an analysis of burden of disease and life expectancy. *The Lancet, 380(9838),* 219-229.

Lee, J.H., O'Keefe, J.H., Lavie, C.J., & Harris, W.S. (2009). Omega-3 fatty acids: cardiovascular benefits, sources and sustainability. *Nature Reviews Cardiology, 6(12),* 753-758.

Leech, R.M., McNaughton, S.A., & Timperio, A. (2014). The clustering of diet, physical activity and sedentary behavior in children and adolescents: a review. *International Journal of Behavioral Nutrition and Physical Activity, 11,* 4.

Levenson, H. (1974). Activism and powerful others: distinctions within the concept of internal-external control. *Journal of Personality Assessment, 38,* 377-383.

Leventhal, H., Musumeci, T.J., & Leventhal, E.A. (2006). Psychological approaches to the connection of health and behavior. *South African Journal of Psychology, 36(4),* 666-682.

Levy, M., & Wang, V. (2013). The framingham heart study and the epidemiology of cardiovascular disease: a historical perspective. *The Lancet, 383(9921)*, 999-1008.

Lim, S.S., Vos, T., Flaxman, A.D., Danaei, G., Shibuya, K., Adair-Rohani, H. … Ezzati, M. (2012). A comparative risk assessment of burden of disease and injury attributable to 67 risk factors and risk factor clusters in 21 regions, 1990–2010: a systematic analysis for the Global Burden of Disease Study 2010. *The Lancet, 380(9859)*, 2224-2260.

Lippke, S., Ziegelmann, J.P., & Schwarzer, R. (2005). Stage-specific adoption and maintenance of physical activity: testing a three-stage model. *Psychology of Sport & Exercise, 6*, 585-603.

Lloyd-Richardson, E.E., Lucero, M.L., DiBello, J.R., Jacobson, A.E., & Wing, R.R. (2008). The relationship between alcohol use, eating habits and weight change in college freshmen. *Eating Behaviors, 9*, 504-508.

Lobelo, F., Duperly, J., & Frank, E. (2009). Physical activity habits of physicians and medical students influence their counseling practices. *British Journal of Sports Medicine, 43*, 89-92.

Lönnroth, K., Williams, G.B., Stadlin, S., Jaramillo, E., & Dye, C. (2008). Alcohol use as a risk factor for tuberculosis – a systematic review. *BMC Public Health, 8*, 289.

Łuszczyńska, A. (2004). *Zmiana zachowań zdrowotnych. Dlaczego dobre chęci nie wystarczają?* Gdańskie Wydawnictwo Psychologiczne, Gdańsk.

Luszczynska, A., & Sutton, S. (2004). Attitudes and expectations. In J. Kerr, R., Weitkunat, & M. Moretti (Eds.). *The ABC of behaviour change. A guide to successful disease prevention and health promotion* (pp. 71-84). Edinburgh, UK: Elsevier.

Mackiewicz M., & Krzyżanowski J. (1981). *Raport o stanie zdrowia społeczeństwa polskiego.* Instytut Medycyny Pracy i Higieny Wsi, Lublin.

MacKinnon, D.P., Fairchild, A.J., & Fritz M.S. (2007). Mediation Analysis. *Annu Rev Psychol., 58*, 593. doi: 10.1146/annurev.psych.58.110405.085542

Maher, J.P., Doerksen, S.E., Elavsky, S., Hyde, A.L., Pincus, A.L., Ram, N., & Conroy, D.E. (2013). A daily analysis of physical activity and satisfaction with life in emerging adults. *Health Psychology, 32(6)*, 647-656.

Malon, A., Deschamps, V., Salanave, B., Vernay, M., Szego, E., Estaquio, C., … Castetbon, K. (2010). Compliance with French nutrition and health program recommendations is strongly associated with socioeconomic characteristics in the general adult population. *Journal of the American Dietetic Association, 110(6)*, 848-856.

Mason, J.O., & Powell, K.E. (1985). Physical activity, behavioral epidemiology, and public health. *Public Health Reports, 100(2)*, 113–115.

Mattei, J., Hu, F.B., & Campos, H. (2011). A higher ratio of beans to white rice is associated with lower cardiometabolic risk factors in Costa Rican adults. *The American Journal of Clinical Nutrition, 94*, 869-876.

Mazurkiewicz, E. (1978). Podstawy wychowania zdrowotnego. In Z.J. Brzeziński, & C.W. Korczak (Eds.) *Higiena i ochrona zdrowia*, Warszawa.

McArdle, N., Hillman, D., Beilin, L., & Watts, G. (2007). Metabolic risk factors for vascular disease in obstructive sleep apnea: a matched controlled study. *The American Journal Critical Care of Medicine, 175(2)*, 190-195.

McAuliffe, W.E., Rohman, M., Breer, P., Wyshak, G., Santangelo, S., & Magnuson, E. (1991). Alcohol use and abuse in random samples of physicians and medical students. *American Journal of Public Health, 81(2)*, 177-182.

McGinnis, J.M., & Foege, W.H. (1993). Actual causes of death in the United States. *The Journal of the American Medical Association, 270*, 2207–2212.

McNerney, J.P., Steven, A., & Deborah L.B. (2007). Self-Reported Health Behaviors of Osteopathic Physicians. *The Journal of the American Osteopathic Association, 107*, 537-546.

Micha, R., Wallace, S.K., & Mozaffarian, D. (2010). Red and processed meat consumption and risk of incident coronary heart disease, stroke, and diabetes mellitus: a systematic review and meta-analysis. *Circulation, 121,* 2271-2283.

Molarius, A., Berglund, K., Eriksson, C., Lambe, M., Nordstro, E., Eriksson, H.G., & Feldman, I. (2006). Socioeconomic conditions, lifestyle factors, and self-rated health among men and women in Sweden. *European Journal of Public Health, 17(2),* 125-133.

Molarius, A., Berglund, K., Eriksson, C., Lambe, M., Nordstrom, E., Eriksson, H.G., & Feldman, I. (2006). Socioeconomic conditions, lifestyle factors, and self-rated health among men and women in Sweden. *European Journal of Public Health, 17(2),* 125-133.

Monograph on TB and tobacco control. (2007). A WHO/The Union. Retrieved from: http://www.who.int/tobacco/resources/publications/tb_tob_control_monograph/en/

Montonen, J., Järvinen, R., Heliövaara, M., & Reunanen, A., Aromaa, A., & Knekt, P. (2005). Food consumption and the incidence of type II diabetes mellitus. *European Journal of Clinical Nutrition, 59,* 441-448.

Mozaffarian, D., Appel, L.J., & Van Horn, L. (2011). Components of a cardioprotective diet: new insights. *Circulation, 123,* 2870-2891.

National Center for Chronic Disease Prevention and Health Promotion. (2007) *Research to Practice Series #1 - Can Eating Fruits and Vegetables Help People Manage Their Weight?* Retrieved from: http://www.cdc.gov/nccdphp/dnpa/nutrition/pdf/rtp_practitioner_10_07.pdf

Nettleton, J.A., Polak, J.F., Tracy, R., Burke, G.L., & Jacobs D.R.Jr (2009). Dietary patterns and incident cardiovascular disease in the Multi-Ethnic Study of Atherosclerosis. *The American Journal of Clinical Nutrition, 90,* 647-654.

Nettleton, J.A., Schulze, M.B., Jiang, R., Jenny, N.S., Burke, G.L., & Jacobs, D.R.Jr (2008). A priori-defined dietary patterns and markers of cardiovascular disease risk in the Multi-Ethnic Study of Atherosclerosis (MESA). *The American Journal of Clinical Nutrition, 88,* 185-194.

Norman, P., Bennett, P., Smith, C., & Murphy, S. (1998). Health locus of control and health behaviour. *Journal of Health Psychology, 3,* 171-180.

OECD. (2012). Health at a Glance: Europe 2012, OECD Publishing. Retrieved from: http://dx.doi.org/10.1787/9789264183896-en

Oken, E., Choi, A.L., Karagas, M.R., Mariën, K., Rheinberger, C.M., Schoeny, R., Sunderland, E., & Korrick, S. (2012). Which fish should I eat? Perspectives influencing fish consumption choices. *Environmental Health Perspectives, 120,* 790-798.

Oreskovich, M.R., Kaups, K.L., Balch, C.M., Hanks, J.B., Satele, D., Sloan, J., ... Shanafelt, T.D. (2012). Prevalence of alcohol use disorders among american surgeons. *Archives of Surgery, 147(2),* 168-174.

Orrow, G., Kinmonth, A.L., Sanderson, S., & Sutton, S. (2012). Effectiveness of physical activity promotion based in primary care: systematic review and meta-analysis of randomised controlled trials. *Britisch Medical Journal 344,* 1389.

Ostrowska, A. (1980). *Elementy kultury zdrowotnej społeczeństwa polskiego.* Ossolineum, Wrocław-Warszawa-Kraków-Gdańsk.

Pan, A., Sun, Q., Bernstein, A.M., Schulze, M.B., Manson, J.E., Willett W.C., & Hu, F.B. (2011). Red meat consumption and risk of type 2 diabetes: 3 cohorts of US adults and an updated meta-analysis. *The American Journal of Clinical Nutrition, 94,* 1088-1096.

Panagiotakos, D., Pitsavos, C., Chrysohoou. C., Palliou, K., Lentzas, I., Skoumas, I., & Stefanadis, C. (2009) Dietary patterns and 5-year incidence of cardiovascular disease: a multivariate analysis of the ATTICA study. *Nutrition, Metabolism and Cardiovascular Diseases 19,* 253.

Pardo, A. (2012). Physical activity level and lifestyle-related risk factors from Catalan physicians. *Preventive Medicine, 55,* 256-257.

Paulik, E., Boka, F., Kertesz, A., Balogh, S., & Nagymajtenyi, L. (2010). Determinants of health-promoting lifestyle behaviour in the rural areas of Hungary. *Health Promotion International, 25(3),* 277-288.

Peluso, M.A.M., & Andrade, L.H.S.G. de. (2005). Physical activity and mental health: the association between exercise and mood. *Clinics, 60(1),* 61-70.

Pereira C.L., Baptista, F., & Infante, P. (2014). Role of physical activity in the occurrence of falls and fall-related injuries in community-dwelling adults over 50 years old. *Disability and Rehabilitation, 36(2),* 117-124.

Petrella, R.J., & Lattanzio, C.N., (2002). Does counseling help patients get active? Systematic review of the literature. *Canadian Family Physician, 48,* 72-80.

Physical activity and health in Europe: evidence for action. (2006). (Eds.) N., Cavill, S., Kahlmeier & F. Racioppi. WHO.

Physical Activity Guidelines Advisory Committee Report. (2008). Department of Health and Human Services, Washington D.C., Retrieved from: http://www.health.gov/paguidelines/Report/pdf/CommitteeReport.pdf

Pliner, P., Bell, R., Hirsch, E.S., & Kinchla, M. (2006). Meal duration mediates the effect of "social facilitation" on eating in humans. *Appetite, 46,*189-198.

Postawy wobec palenia papierosów. (2012). Raport BS/107/2012 Centrum Badania Opinii Społecznej, Warszawa Retrieved from: http://www.cbos.pl/SPISKOM.POL/2012/K_107_12.PDF

Powell, K.E., Paluch, A.E., & Blair, S.N. (2011). Physical activity for health: What kind? How much? How intense? On top of what? *Annual Review of Public Health, 32,* 349-365.

Poździoch, S.J. (1975). Socjologiczna problematyka zachowań zdrowotnych. In J. Indulski (Ed.) *Materiały do ćwiczeń z medycyny społecznej.* Wybrane zagadnienia socjologii medycyny. Łódź.

Preacher, K.J., & Hayes, A.F. (2008). Asymptotic and resampling strategies for assessing and comparing indirect effects in multiple mediator models. *Behavior Research Methods, 40,* 879-891.

Principles of Proper Nutrition. (2009). Instytut Zywienia i Zywności. Retrieved from: http://www.izz.waw.pl/pl/zasady-prawidowego-ywienia#c

Prochaska, J.J. (2008). Multiple health behaviour research represents the future of preventive medicine. *Preventive Medicine, 46,* 281–285.

Prochaska, J.J. (2011). A review of multiple health behavior change interventions for primary prevention. *American Journal Of Lifestyle Medicine, 5(3),* 208-221.

Prochaska, J.O. & DiClemente, C.C. (1983). Stages and processes of self-change in smoking: toward an integrative model of change. *Journal of Consulting and Clinical Psychology, 5,* 390–395.

Prochaska, J.O. (2008). Multiple health behavior research represents the future of preventive medicine. *Preventive Medicine, 46(3),* 281-285.

Prochaska, J.O., DiClemente, C.C., & Norcross, J.C. (1992). In search of how people change: applications to addictive behaviors. *American Psychologist, 47,* 1102-1114.

Pronk, N.P., Anderson, L.H., Crain, A.L., Martinson, B.C., O'Connor, P.J., Sherwood, N.E., & Whitebird, R.R. (2004). Meeting recommendations for multiple healthy lifestyle factors. Prevalence, clustering, and predictors among adolescent, adult, and senior health plan members. *American Journal of Preventive Medicine, 27,* 25-33.

Puchalski, K. (1989a). Pojęcie zachowań związanych ze zdrowiem. In: *Socjologia zdrowia i medycyny. Materiały konserwatorium 1986-88,* IFIS PAN, Warszawa.

Puchalski, K. (1989b). Zachowania zdrowotne. Kontrowersje związane z użyciem pojęcia. *Zdrowie Publiczne, 100(1).*

Puchalski, K. (1990). Zachowania związane ze zdrowiem jako przedmiot nauk socjologicznych. Uwagi wokół pojęcia. In A. Gniazdowski (Ed.). *Zachowania zdrowotne. Zagadnienie teoretyczne, próba charakterystyki zachowań zdrowotnych społeczeństwa polskiego.* (pp. 47-56). Instytut Medycyny Pracy im. Prof.dr med. Jerzego Nofera, Łódź.

Puchalski, K. (1997). *Zdrowie w świadomości społecznej.* Instytut Medycyny Pracy im. Prof.dr med. Jerzego Nofera, Krajowe Centrum Promocji Zdrowia w Miejscu Pracy, Łódź.

Puchalski, K. (2000). Promocja zdrowia w dużych zakładach pracy w Polsce. Aktualny stan i niektóre uwarunkowania. *Promocja Zdrowia, Nauki Społeczne i Medycyna, 7(19),* 66-87.

Puciato, D., Rozpara, M., Mynarski, W., Łoś, A., & Królikowska, B. (2013). Physical activity of adult residents of Katowice and selected determinants of their occupational status and socio-economic characteristics. *Medycyna Pracy, 64(5),* 649-657.

Puddester D., Flynn L.,& Cohen J. (2009). *CanMEDS physician health guide: A practical handbook for physician health and well-being.* Ottawa: The Royal College of Physicians and Surgeons of Canada.

Rasińska, R., & Nowakowska, I. (2012). Smoking among students – the comparison of author's own investigations with literature. *Przegląd Lekarski, 69,* 888-892.

Rehm, J., Mathers, C., Popova, S., Thavorncharoensap, M., Teerawattananon, Y., & Patra, J. (2009). Global burden of disease and injury and economic cost attributable to alcohol use and alcohol-use disorders. *The Lancet, 373,* 2223-2233.

Rehm, J., Room, R., Kathryn, G., Monteiro, M., Gmel, G., & Sempos, C.T. (2003). The relationship of average volume of alcohol consumption and patterns of drinking to burden of disease: an overview. *Addiction, 98(9),* 1209-1228.

Reilly, J.M., (2007). Are obese physicians effective at providing healthy lifestyle counseling? *American Family Physician, 75(5),* 738-741.

Reimers, C.D., Knapp, G., & Reimers A.K. (2012). Does Physical Activity Increase Life Expectancy? A Review of the Literature. *Journal of Aging Research, 2012.*

Reynolds, K., Lewis, B., Nolen, J.D.L., Kinney, G.L., Sathya, B., & He, J. (2003). Alcohol consumption and risk of stroke. A meta-analysis. *The Journal of the American Medical Association, 289(5),* 579-588.

Rice, B.H., Quann, E.E., & Miller, G.D. (2013). Meeting and exceeding dairy recommendations: effects of dairy consumption on nutrient intakes and risk of chronic disease. *Nutrition Reviews, 71(4),* 209-223.

Rogers, E.M. (1995). *Diffusion of innovations (4th edition).* New York: The Free Press.

Rohrmann, S., Overvad, K., Bueno-de-Mesquita, H.B., Jakobsen, M.U., Egeberg, R., Tjønneland, A., ... Linseisen, J. (2013). Meat consumption and mortality - results from the european prospective investigation into cancer and nutrition. *BMC Medicine, 11,* 63.

Ronksley, P.E., Brien, S.E., Turner, B.J., Mukamal, K.J., & Ghali, W.A. (2011). Association of alcohol consumption with selected cardiovascular disease outcomes: a systematic review and meta-analysis. *BMJ, 2011,* 342.

Rosenstock, I.M. (1966). Why people use health services. *Milbank Memorial Fund Quarterly, 83(4),* 1-32.

Rosta, J., & Aasland, O.G. (2013). Changes in alcohol drinking patterns and their consequences among norwegian doctors from 2000 to 2010: a longitudinal study based on national samples. *Alcohol and Alcoholism, 48(1),* 99-106.

Rotter, J.B. (1966). Generalized expectancies for internal and external control of reinforcement. *Psychological Monographs: General Applied, 80(1),* 1-28.

Rucker, D.D., Preacher, K.J., Tormala, Z.L., & Petty, R.E. (2011). Mediation analysis in social psychology: Current practices and new recommendations. *Social and Personality Psychology Compass, 5/6,* 359-371.

Ruiz-Canela, M., & Martínez-González, M.A. (2011). Olive oil in the primary prevention of cardio-vascular disease. *Maturitas, 68(3),* 245-250.

Sakamaki, R., Toyama, K., Amamoto, R., Liu, C.J., Shinfuku, N. (2005). Nutritional knowledge, food habits and health attitude of Chinese university students: a cross sectional study. *Nutrition Journal, 4(4).*

Salas-Salvadó, J., Bulló, M., Babio, N., Martínez-gonzález, M.Á., Ibarrola-jurado, N., Basora, J., ... Ros, E. (2011). Reduction in the incidence of type 2 diabetes with the mediterranean diet results of the PREDIMED-Reus nutrition intervention randomized trial. *Diabetes Care January, 34(1),* 14-19.

Samieri, C., Féart, C., Proust-Lima, C., Peuchant, E., Tzourio, C., Stapf, C., ... Barberger-Gateau, P. (2011). Olive oil consumption, plasma oleic acid, and stroke incidence. *The Three-City Study Neurology 77(5),* 418-425.

Schmid, D., & Leitzmann, M.F. (2014). Association between physical activity and mortality among breast cancer and colorectal cancer survivors: a systematic review and meta-analysis. *Annals Of Oncology, 25(7),* 1293-1311.

Schuit, A., van Loon, J., Tijhuis, M., & Ocke´, M. (2002). Clustering of lifestyle risk factors in a general adult population. *Preventive Medicine, 35,* 219–224.

Schwarzer, R. (2001). Social-cognitive factors in changing health-related behaviors. *Current Directions in Psychological Science, 10(2),* 47-51.

Schwarzer, R. (2008). Modeling health behavior change: how to predict and modify the adoption and maintenance of health behaviors. *Applied Psychology, 57(1),* 1-29.

Schwarzer, R., & Renner, B. (2000a). *Health-Specific Self-Efficacy Scales.* Retrieved from: http://userpage.fu-berlin.de/~health/healself.pdf

Schwarzer, R., & Renner, B. (2000b). Social-cognitive predictors of health behavior: action self-efficacy and coping self-efficacy. *Health-Psychology, 19,* 487-495.

Sebo, P., Gallacchi, M.B., Goehring, C., Künzi, B., & Bovier, P.A. (2007). Use of tobacco and alcohol by Swiss primary care physicians: a cross-sectional survey. *BMC Public Health, 7,* 5.

Shaikh, A.R., Yaroch, A.L., Nebeling, L., Yeh, M.C, & Resnicow, K. (2008). Psychosocial predictors of fruit and vegetable consumption in adults: a review of the literature. *American Journal of Preventive Medicine, 34,* 535-543.

Shield K.D., Kehoe, T., Gmel, G., Rehm M.X., & Rehm, J. (2012). Societal burden of alcohol. In P. Anderson, L. Moller, G. Galea (Eds.) *Alcohol in the European Union. Consumption, harm and policy approaches.* (pp. 10-26) Copenhagen, WHO Regional Office for Europe

Shrout, P. E., & Bolger, N. (2002). Mediation in experimental and nonexperimental studies: new procedures and recommendations. *Psychological Methods, 7(4),* 422-445.

Siemińska, A., Jassem, J.M., Uherek, M., Wilanowski, T., Nowak, R., & Jassem, E. (2006). Postawy wobec palenia tytoniu wśród studentów pierwszego roku medycyny. *Pneumonologia i Alergologia Polska, 74,* 377-382.

Sinha, R., Cross, A.J., Graubard, B.I., Leitzmann, M.F., & Schatzkin, A. (2009). Meat intake and mortality: a prospective study of over half a million people. *Archives of Internal Medicine, 169,* 562-571.

Słońska Z. (2002). Promocja zdrowia w Polsce. Ograniczenia systemowe. In W. Piątkowski & A. Titkow (Eds.), *W stronę socjologii zdrowia* (pp. 259-277), Wydawnictwo Uniwersytetu Marii Curie Skłodowskiej, Lublin.

Słońska, Z., & Misiuna, M. (1993). *Promocja zdrowia. Słownik podstawowych terminów.* Agencja Promo-Lider, Warszawa.

Smith, D.R., & Leggat, P.A. (2007). An international review of tobacco smoking in the medical profession: 1974–2004. *BMC Public Health, 7,* 115.

Smith, K.J., Sanderson, K., McNaughton, S.A., Gall, S.L., Dwyer, T., & Venn A.J. (2014). Longitudinal associations between fish consumption and depression in young adults. *American Journal of Epidemiology, 179(10),* 1228-1235.

Smolinska, K., & Paluszkiewicz, P. (2010). Risk of colorectal cancer in relation to frequency and total amount of red meat consumption. Systematic review and meta-analysis. *Archives of Medical Science, 6,* 605-610.

Snyderman, R., & Yoediono, Z. (2008). Perspective: prospective health care and the role of academic medicine: lead, follow, or get out of the way. *Academic Medicine, 83,* 707-714.

Soedamah-Muthu, S.S., Ding, E.L., Al-Delaimy, W.K., Hu, F.B., Engberink, M.F., Willett, W.C., & Geleijnse, J.M. (2011). Milk and dairy consumption and incidence of cardiovascular diseases and all-cause mortality: dose-response meta-analysis of prospective cohort studies. *The American Journal of Clinical Nutrition, 93,* 158-171.

Sokołowska M.(1968). Zastosowanie socjologii w medycynie. In A. Podgórecki (Ed.), *Socjotechnika. Praktyczne zastosowania socjologii.* PWN, Warszawa.

Sonstroem, R. (1984). Exercise and self-esteem. *Sport Science Review, 12,* 123-155.

Special Eurobarometer Research 412 (2014). Sport and physical activity. Brussels, European Commission, Retrived from: http://ec.europa.eu/public_opinion/archives/eb_ special_419_400_en.htm

Sport and Physical Activity. (2010). Eurobarometer 72.3, TNS Opinion & Social, Belgium

Stan zagrożenia epidemią palenia tytoniu w Polsce. (2009). WHO Regional Office for Europe.

Status Report On Alcohol And Health in 35 European Countries. (2013). WHO Regional Office for Europe. Retrieved from: http://www.euro.who.int/__data/assets/pdf_file/0017/190430/ Status-Report-on-Alcohol-and-Health-in-35-European-Countries.pdf?ua=1

Steptoe, A., & Wardle, J. (2001). Locus of control and health behavior revisited: A multivariate analysis of young adults from 18 countries. *British Journal of Psychology, 92(4),* 659-672.

Steptoe, A., & Wardle, J. (2001a). Health behaviour, risk awareness and emotional well-being in students from Eastern Europe and Western Europe. *Social Science & Medicine, 53,* 1621–1630.

Steptoe, A., & Wardle, J. (2001b). Locus of control and health behaviour revisited: A multivariate analysis of young adults from 18 countries. *British Journal of Psychology, 92,* 659–672.

Stożek, E. (2010). O czym mówi efekt standardowy? Retrieved from: http://www.ptde.org/file.php/1/ Archiwum/XI/57.pdf

Strecher, V.J., DeVellis, B.M., Becker, M.H., & Rosenstock, I.M. (1986). The role of self-efficacy in achieving health behavior change. *Health Education Quarterly, 13,* 73–92.

Stretcher, V., Wang, C., Derry, H., Wildenhaus, K., & Johnson, C. (2002). Tailored interventions for multiple risk behaviors. *Health Education Research, 17,* 619–626.

Sutton, S. (2000). Interpreting cross-sectional data on stages of change. *Psychology & Health, 15(2),* 163-171.

Sutton, S. (2002). Using social cognition models to develop health behaviour interventions: Problems and assumptions. In D. Rutter & L. Quine (Eds), *Changing health behaviour: Intervention and research with social cognition models.* (pp. 193-208). Maidenhead, BRK, England: Open University Press.

Svetkey, P., Simons-Morton, D., Vollmer, M., Appel, J., Conlin, R., Ryan, D., Ard, J., & Kennedy, M. (1999). Effects of dietary patterns on blood pressure: subgroup analysis of the Dietary Approaches to Stop Hypertension (DASH) randomized clinical trial. *Archive of Internal Medicine, 159,* 285-293.

Taha, E.A., Ez-Aldin, A.M., Sayed, S.K., Ghandour, N.M., & Mostafa, T. (2012). Effect of smoking on sperm vitality, DNA integrity, seminal oxidative stress, zinc in fertile men. *Urology, 80(4),* 822-825.

The Helsinki Statement on Health in All Policies, (2013). The 8th Global Conference on Health Promotion, Helsinki, Finland, 10-14 June 2013

The Ottawa Charter for Health Promotion (1986). First International Conference on Health Promotion, Ottawa

The smoker's body. Tobacco Free Initiative, (2004). Retrieved from: http://www.who.int/tobacco.

Theory at a Glance A Guide For Health Promotion Practice. (2005), U.S. Department Of Health And Human Services Nih Publication No. 05-3896. Retrieved from: http://www.cancer.gov/ cancertopics/cancerlibrary/theory.pdf

Thibaud, M., Bloch, F., Tournoux-Facon, C., Brèque, C., Rigaud, A., Dugué, B., & Kemoun, G. (2012). Impact of physical activity and sedentary behaviour on fall risks in older people: a systematic review and meta-analysis of observational studies. *European Reviews of Aging & Physical Activity, 9(1),* 5.

Thompson, M.D., Mensack, M.M., Jiang, W., Zhu, Z., Lewis, M.R., McGinley, J.N., ... Thompson, H.J. (2012). Cell signaling pathways associated with a reduction in mammary cancer burden by dietary common bean (Phaseolus vulgaris L.). *Carcinogenesis, 33(1),* 226-232.

Titkow, A. (1983), *Zachowania i postawy wobec zdrowia i choroby. Studium warszawskie.* PWN, Warszawa.

Tobacco fact sheet No. 339. (2014). Geneva: World Health Organization; Retrieved from: http://www.who.int/mediacentre/factsheets/fs339/en

Tobacco. Special Eurobarometer 332. (2010). Wave 72.3, TNS Opinion & Social. Belgium

Tobiasz-Adamczyk, B. (1998). *Wybrane elementy socjologii zdrowia i choroby.* Kraków.

Troiano, R.P., Berrigan, D., Dodd, K.W., Masse, L.C., Tilert, T., & McDowell, M. (2008). Physical activity in the United States measured by accelerometer. *Medicine & Science in Sports & Exercise, 40(1).*

Tsai, J., Ford, E.S., Li, C., Zhao, G., Pearson, W.S., & Balluz, L.S. (2010). Multiple healthy behaviors and optimal self-rated health: findings from the 2007 behavioral risk factor surveillance system survey. *Preventive Medicine, 51(3-4),* 268-274.

U.S. EPA (Environmental Protection Agency). (2004). FDA/EPA Consumer Advisory: What You Need to Know about Mercury in Fish and Shellfish. Retrieved from: http://www.epa.gov/ost/fishadvice/factsheet.html

Van Zundert, R.M., Ferguson, S.G., Shiffman, S., Engels, R.C.M.E. (2010). Dynamic effects of self-efficacy on smoking lapses and relapse among adolescents. *Health Psychology, 29(3),* 246-254.

Velicer, W.F., DiClemente, C.C., Rossi, J.S., Prochaska, J.O. (1990). Relapse situations and self-efficacy: An integrative model. *Addictive Behaviors, 15,* 271-283.

Waist Circumference and Waist–Hip Ratio. (2011). Report of a WHO expert consultation. Geneva, WHO

Wallston, K. A., Wallston, B.S. & DeVellis, R. (1978). Development of the multidimensional health locus of control (MHLC) scales. *Health Education Monographs, 6,* 160-170.

Wang, S., Meckling, K.A., Marcone, M.F., Kakuda, Y., & Tsao, R. (2011). Synergistic, additive, and antagonistic effects of food mixtures on total antioxidant capacities. *Journal of Agricultural and Food Chemistry, 59(3),* 960-968.

Warburton, D.E.R, Nicol C.W., & Bredin, S.S.D. (2006). Health benefits of physical activity: the evidence. *CMAJ, 174(6),* 801-809.

Warburton, D.E.R., Charlesworth, S., Ivey, A., Nettlefold, L., & Bredin, S.S.D. (2010). A systematic review of the evidence for Canada's physical activity guidelines for adults. *International Journal of Behavioral Nutrition and Physical Activity, 7(1),* 39.

Wardle, J., & Steptoe, A. (2003). Socioeconomic differences in attitudes and beliefs about healthy lifestyles. *Journal of Epidemiology & Community Health, 57,* 440-443.

Weinstein, N. D., & Sandman, P. M. (2002). The Precaution Adoption Process Model and its application. In R.J. DiClemente, R. A. Crosby, & M.C. Kegler (Eds.) *Emerging theories in health promotion practice and research. Strategies for improving public health.* (pp. 16-39). San Francisco: Jossey-Bass.

Weinstein, N.D., Sandman, P.M., & Blalock, S.J. (2008). The precaution adoption process model. In K. Glanz, B. K. Rimer, and K. Viswanath (Eds.), *Health Behavior and Health Education.* 4th. ed. (pp. 123–147). San Francisco: Jossey-Bass,.

White, H.R., McMorris, B.J., Catalano, R.F., Fleming, C.B., Haggerty, K.P., & Abbott, R.D. (2006). Increases in alcohol and marijuana use during the transition out of high school into emerging adulthood: the effects of leaving home, going to college, and high school protective factors. *Journal of Studies on Alcohol and Drugs, 67(6),* 810-822.

WHO expert consultation. Appropriate body-mass index for Asian populations and its implications for policy and intervention strategies (2004). *The Lancet*, 157-163.

WHO Framework Convention on Tobacco Control. (2003). Geaneva: Health Organization, Retrieved from: http://www.who.int/fctc/text_download/en/

WHO Global Report: Mortality Attributable to Tobacco. (2012). Geneva: World Health Organization. Retrieved from: http://whqlibdoc.who.int/publications/2012/9789241564434_eng.pdf

WHO report on the global tobacco epidemic 2013: enforcing bans on tobacco advertising, promotion and sponsorship (2013). Geneva: World Health Organization. Retrieved from: http://www.who.int/tobacco/global_report/access_form/en/index.html

WHO. Obesity: preventing and managing the global epidemic. (2000). Report of a WHO Consultation. WHO Technical Report Series 894. Geneva: World Health Organization

WHO. Physical status: the use and interpretation of anthropometry (1995). Report of a WHO Expert Committee. WHO Technical Report Series 854. Geneva: World Health Organization

Wiefferink, C.H., Peters, L., Hoekstra, F., Dam, G.T., Buijs, G.J., & Paulussen, T.G.W.M. (2006). Clustering of health-related behaviors and their determinants: possible consequences for school health interventions. *Prevention Science, 7(2).*

Willett, W.C. & Stampfer, M.J. (2006). Rebuilding the food pyramid. *Scientific American, 16,* 12-21.

Willett, W.C. (2012). Dietary fats and coronary heart disease. *Journal of Internal Medicine, 272(1).*

Willett, W.C., Skerrett, P.J. & Giovannucci, E.L. (2005) *Eat, drink, and be healthy: The Harvard Medical School Guide to Healthy Eating.* Simon & Schuster.

World Cancer Research Fund/American Institute for Cancer Research. (2007). *Food, Nutrition, Physical Activity, and the Prevention of Cancer: a Global Perspective.* Washington DC: American Institute for Cancer Research

Woronowicz, B.T. (2010). Medice, cura te ipsum. *Gazeta Lekarska 6-7,* 22-23.

Wu, S., Wang, R., Zhao, Y., Ma, X., Wu, M., Yan, X., & He, J. (2013). The relationship between self-rated health and objective health status: a population-based study. *BMC Public Health, 13,* 320.

Wu, S., Wang, R., Zhao, Y., Ma, X., Wu, M., Yan, X., & He, Y. (2013). The relationship between self-rated health and objective health status: a population-based study. *BMC Public Health, 13(320).*

Ye, E.Q., Chacko, S.A., Chou, E.L., Kugizaki, M., & Liu, S. (2012). Greater whole-grain intake is associated with lower risk of type 2 diabetes, cardiovascular disease, and weight gain. *The Journal of Nutrition, 142,* 1304-1313.

Ye, Q.E., Chacko, S.A., Chou, E.L., Kugizaki, M., & Liu, S. (2012). Greater whole-grain intake is associated with lower risk of type 2 diabetes, cardiovascular disease, and weight gain. *The Journal of Nutrition Nutritional Epidemiology, 142,* 1304-1313.

Zachowania i nawyki żywieniowe Polaków (2010). Centrum Badania Opinii Społecznej, Warszawa. Retrieved from: http://badanie.cbos.pl/details.asp?q=a1&id=4389

Zhao, X., Lynch, J. G., Jr, & Chen, Q. (2010). Reconsidering Baron and Kenny: Myths and truths about mediation analysis. *Journal of Consumer Research, 37,* 197-206.

Ziemska, B. (2012). *Stan zdrowia pracowników Uniwersytetu Medycznego im. Karola Marcinkowskiego w Poznaniu.* Praca doktorska. Promotor Marcinkowski, J.T., Poznań.

Ziemska, B., & Marcinkowski, J.T. (2010). Stan zdrowia pracowników Uniwersytetu Medycznego w Poznaniu. *Problemy Higieny i Epidemiologii, 91(1),* 54-56.

Zysnarska, M., Bernad, D., & Kara, A., (2007). Palenie papierosów przez pielęgniarki zatrudnione na oddziałach onkologicznych w aspekcie realizowanych zadań edukacyjnych, *Przegląd Lekarski, 10,* 842-844

List of Figures

List of Tables

Index

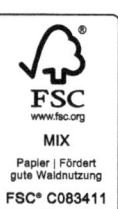

Zeitfracht Medien GmbH
Ferdinand-Jühlke-Straße 7
99095 Erfurt, Deutschland
produktsicherheit@kolibri360.de